WILLIAM ALEXANDER HAMMOND

SPIRITUALISM

AND

ALLIED CAUSES AND CONDITIONS

OF

NERVOUS DERANGEMENT

Elibron Classics
www.elibron.com

Elibron Classics series.

ISBN 1-4021-9425-0 (paperback)
ISBN 1-4021-1039-1 (hardcover)

This Elibron Classics Replica Edition is an unabridged facsimile of the edition published in 1876 by H.K. Lewis, London.

SPIRITUALISM

AND

ALLIED CAUSES AND CONDITIONS

OF

NERVOUS DERANGEMENT

BY

WILLIAM A. HAMMOND, M.D.

Professor of Diseases of the Mind and Nervous System in the Medical Department of the University of the City of New York, etc.

"Ratio quasi quædam lux lumenque vitæ."—Cicero.

ILLUSTRATED.

LONDON

H. K. LEWIS

136 Gower Street

1876

I DEDICATE THIS BOOK TO ALL,

FEW THOUGH THEY BE,

WHO ARE FREE FROM SUPERSTITION.

PREFACE.

"THE Physics and Physiology of Spiritualism," a little book based upon an article contributed to the *North American Review*, having for several years been out of print, I have taken the opportunity presented by the demand for a new edition to reform the work, and to extend it very far beyond its original limits. In so doing I have not only re-written and amplified the remarks on Spiritualism, but have included within the scope of the present volume several other subjects, not only analogous in their scientific relations to the discussion in question, but which are in themselves, perhaps, still more interesting to the general reader.

Throughout, my object has been to strip from the basis of fact, which almost always exists, the network of error which ignorance, credulity and superstition have woven around it. In making this attempt I have endeavored to avoid saying a word which could be tortured into an expression of disrespect for true and rational religion of any kind, especially for the fundamental beliefs of Christianity to which the civilized world owes so much. But for the faith, whether spiritualistic or mesmeric; whether medical or theological; whether orthodox or heterodox; whether Christian or Pagan; whether Protestant or Roman Catholic, which seeks to bolster itself up by so-called supernatural phenomena, or by alleged miraculous interpositions of the Deity in its behalf, I have not hesitated to speak with entire frankness and directness.

And I confess that for the religion which is mainly based

upon emotion I have no great respect. It is generally as fleeting as the inconstant feeling from which it arises, while leaving behind it mental and nervous disorders often of life-long duration. The "Outpouring of the Spirit of God"—an expression which would be blasphemous if it were not the result of ignorance—is too often, to the physician's perception, only another name for epilepsy, chorea, catalepsy, ecstasy, hysteria or insanity.

This book is not therefore written in the interest of science against religion. Its aim is altogether different. Indeed there can be no conflict between pure science and pure religion; for the one is truth and the other is faith in the truth. But between science and the distorted facts, the misinterpreted phenomena, the gross and senseless delusions with which individuals have from time to time bedaubed the features of natural religion, warfare is perpetual, and in that contest the position of this little work is not doubtful.

43 WEST 54th ST., NEW YORK,
MAY 1, 1876.

CONTENTS.

CHAPTER I.

CHAPTER II.

CHAPTER III.

CHAPTER IV.

CHAPTER V.

CHAPTER VI.

CHAPTER XIII.

CHAPTER XIV.

SPIRITUALISM,

AND

ALLIED CAUSES OF NERVOUS DERANGEMENT.

CHAPTER I.

SOME OF THE CAUSES WHICH LEAD TO A BELIEF IN SPIRITUALISM—SENSORIAL DECEPTION.

THERE is an inherent tendency in the mind of man to ascribe to supernatural agencies those events the causes of which are beyond his knowledge; and this is especially the case with the normal and morbid phenomena which are manifested in his own person. But, as his intellect becomes more thoroughly trained, and as science advances in its developments, the range of his credulity becomes more and more circumscribed, his doubts are multiplied, and he at length reaches that condition of "healthy skepticism" which allows of no belief without the proof. Thus he does not now credit the existence of an *archæus* dwelling in the stomach and presiding over its function, for he knows by experiment that digestion is a purely physical process, which can be as well performed in a teacup, with a little pepsin and dilute chlorhydric acid, as in the stomach with the gastric juice; he does not now believe that the bodies of lunatics, epileptics, and hysterical women, are inhabited by devils and demons, for he has ascertained by observation that the abnormal conditions present in such persons can be accounted for by material derangements of the organs or functions of the system. He has learned to doubt, and, therefore to reason better ; he makes experiments, collects facts, does not begin to theorize until his data are sufficient, and then is careful that his theories do not extend beyond the foundation of certainty, or at least of probability, upon which he builds.

But there have always been, and probably always will be, individuals whose love for the marvellous is so great, and whose logical powers are so small, as to render them susceptible of entertaining any belief, no matter how preposterous it may be ; and others more numerous, who, staggered by facts which they cannot understand, accept any hypothesis which may be offered as an explanation, rather than confess their ignorance.

The real and fraudulent phenomena of what is called spiritualism are of such a character as to make a profound impression upon the credulous and the ignorant ; and both these classes have accordingly been active in spreading the most exaggerated ideas relative to matters which are either absurdly false or not so very astonishing when viewed by the cold light of science. Such persons have, probably, from a very early age, believed in the materiality of spirits ; and having very little knowledge of the forces inherent in their own bodies, have no difficulty in ascribing occurrences, which do not accord with their experience, to the agency of disembodied individuals whom they imagine to be circulating through the world. In this respect they resemble those savages who regard the burning-lens, the mirror, and other things which produce unfamiliar effects, as being animated by deities. Their minds are decidedly fetish-worshipping in character, and are scarcely, in this respect, of a more elevated type than that of the Congo negro who endows the rocks and trees with higher mental attributes than he claims for himself.

Then it is possible for the most careful and experienced judgment to be deceived by false sensorial impressions of real objects, or by non-existing images created by the mind. In the first case a gleam of moonlight passes for a ghost, the stump of a tree becomes a robber, and the rustling of leaves blown by the wind is imagined to be the whispering of voices. No one possesses an absolute perfection of sensation, and thus things are never seen, or heard, or smelt, or tasted, or felt exactly as they exist. In the dark, or in the uncertain light of the moon, or of artificial illumination, the liability to self-deception is very much increased; and if, in addition to the defect of light, there are continual sounds and other means of engaging the attention, it is exceedingly easy to induce sensorial confusion and thus to impose upon the intellect.

The so-called mediums know very well the advantages to be derived from darkness, musical sounds and other ways of diverting the senses from the real object they have in view, and every magician, conjurer, and legerdemainist makes use of the same means as a special element in the success of his tricks.

Thus the medium, or the honest prestidigitateur tells the subject who is to be deceived that he must concentrate his mind on his great-grandmother, for instance, and that in a few minutes she will make her appearance. If the victim be weak of intellect and highly impressionable, it is fully within the range of probability that no further efforts will be required from the worker of the pretended miracle. The apparition of the deceased ancestor will be present to the eyes of the descendant. But even if he be gifted with an ordinary amount of cerebral development the concentration of his attention upon a single subject, places him in the most favorable possible condition to be deceived by any manœuvres of the medium or magician, to be still further guided by his suggestions, or to misinterpret real occurrences which may be produced.

As regards purely imaginary images—that is, images not based on any sensorial impression—the trouble is in the brain. An excess or deficiency of blood circulating through this organ, or a morbid alteration of its quality, such as is induced by alcohol, opium, belladonna, and other similar substances, will often lead to hallucinations. Those of De Quincey, Coleridge, and other opium-eaters, are well known, and several striking instances have come under my own notice.

Various mental emotions act in a like manner by their influence in deranging the cerebral circulation. A young lady who had overtasked her mind at school, was thrown thereby into a semi-hysterical condition during which she saw spectres of various kinds which passed and repassed rapidly before her all day long. Everything at which she looked appeared to her of enormous size. A head, for instance, seemed to be several feet in diameter, and little children looked like giants. When I took out my watch while examining her pulse, she remarked that it was as large as the wheel of a carriage. Sauvages refers to a somewhat similar case, in which a young woman, suffering from epilepsy, saw dreadful images, and to whom real objects appeared to be greatly magnified. A fly seemed as large as a chicken, and a chicken equalled an ox in size.

Physical causes, calculated to increase the amount of blood in the brain or to alter its quality, may give rise to hallucinations of various kinds. A gentleman under the professional charge of the writer, can always cause the appearance of images by tying a handkerchief moderately tight around his neck; and there is one form which is always the first to come and the last to disappear. It consists of a male figure clothed in the costume worn in England three hundred years ago, and bearing a striking resemblance to the portraits of Sir Walter Raleigh. This figure not only imposes on the sight, but also on the hearing; for questions put to it are answered promptly, and with much more intellectual force than those addressed to the so called "spirits." How easy would it be for the gentleman subject to this hallucination, were he a believer in spiritualism, and less intelligent, to imagine that his visitor was a spirit, and that he held converse with the real Sir Walter Raleigh!

A similar instance is related in Nicholson's Journal.* "I know a gentleman," he states, "in the vigor of life, who, in my opinion, is not exceeded by any one in acquired knowledge and originality of deep research; and who for nine months in succession was always visited by a figure of the same man, threatening to destroy him, at the time of his going to rest. It appeared upon his lying down, and instantly disappeared when he resumed the erect position." The explanation here is very simple. The recumbent position facilitated the flow of blood to the brain, and at the same time tended, in a measure, to retard its exit. Hence the appearance of the figure was due to the resulting congestion. As soon as the gentleman rose

* Vol. vi.. p. 166.

from bed the reverse conditions existed, the congestion disappeared and the apparition went with it.

The other senses may be individually affected, or may participate in the general disturbance. It is by no means uncommon for physicians to meet with cases in which either the smell, the taste, or the touch is the subject of hallucinatory impressions. A gentleman recently under the care of the writer, is constantly under the idea that he smells turpentine. For a time the conviction was so strong that he could not resist the impulse to search for the origin of this odor, but as he was never once rewarded with success in his efforts, he gradually came to regard the cause as entirely subjective. Still he is never free, except during sleep, from the smell of turpentine in his nostrils.

Another has the sensation of touch on the top of his head so deranged, that he is sure there is something pressing hard upon his scalp. Even the correction which he is enabled to give through the ends of his fingers does not suffice to eradicate the idea. He resists, as well as he is able, for several minutes at a time, and then, goaded on by the sensation "that there is something there," he raises his hand to remove it, only to be undeceived for a brief period.

Mayo * relates the case of a Herr von Baczko, already subject to hallucinations, his right side weak from paralysis, his right eye blind, and the vision of the left imperfect, who, while one evening engaged in translating a pamphlet into Polish, suddenly felt a poke in his back. He turned round and discovered that it proceeded from a negro or Egyptian boy, apparently

* Lessons on the truths contained in Popular Superstitions, Frankfort-on-the-Maine, 1849, p. 47.

about twelve years of age. Although convinced that the whole was an hallucination, he thought it best to knock the apparition down, when he felt that it offered a sensible resistance. The boy then attacked him on the other side and gave his left arm a peculiarly disagreeable twist, when Baczko again pushed him off. The negro continued to visit him constantly during four months, preserving the same appearance and remaining tangible, then he came seldomer, and finally appearing as a brown colored apparition with an owl's head, he took his leave.

The fact that multitudes may be simultaneously impressed with the same belief, is no guaranty that this belief is founded on reality. A great many otherwise sensible people have been convinced that the blood of St. Januarius periodically undergoes liquefaction; yet those, whose education and habits of thought teach them to look upon such so-called miracles with distrust, are not brought to accept the truth of the legend, because many thousands of other persons have received it in full faith.

Josephus * states that "a few days after the feast of the Passover, on the twenty-first day of the month Artemisius, a certain prodigious and incredible phenomenon appeared. I suppose the account of it would seem to be a fable were it not related by those that saw it, and were not the events that followed it of so considerable a nature as to deserve such signals; for, before sun-setting, chariots, and troops of soldiers in their armor, were seen running about among the clouds, and surrounding of cities. Moreover, at that feast, which we call Pen-

* The works of Flavius Josephus; translated by William Whiston, A.M., Professor of Mathematics in the University of Cambridge. The Wars of the Jews, chap. vi., book vi.

tecost, as the priests were going by night into the inner court of the temple, as their custom was, to perform their sacred ministrations, they said that in the first place they felt a quaking and heard a great noise, and after that they heard a great sound as of a great multitude saying, 'Let us remove hence.'"

The army of Constantine saw the cross in the sky, with the legend "*In hoc signo vinces.*" The Crusaders were often witnesses of like imaginary prodigies. At the battle of Antioch "a squadron was seen to descend from the summit of the mountains, preceded by three horsemen, clothed in white and covered with shining armor. 'Behold,' cried Bishop Adelman, 'the heavenly succor which was promised to you; Heaven declares for the Christians; the holy martyrs St. George, Demetrius and Theodore come to fight for you.' Immediately all eyes were turned towards the celestial legions. A new ardor inspired the Christians, who were persuaded that God himself was coming to their aid."*

Ferrier † quotes an Italian writer to the effect that upon one occasion, in the streets of Florence, a crowd was assembled earnestly beholding the image of an angel hovering in the sky. A philosopher explained to the excited multitude that the circumstance was a deception caused by a mist which partially covered the dome of a church, surmounted by the gilded figure of an angel, in such a manner as to allow the image to be illuminated by the rays of the sun. Without the presence of this sensible man the event would have passed for a supernatural appearance.

It is only necessary to refer to the writers of three or four

* Michaud's History of the Crusades. Translated from the French by W. Robson, London, 1852. Vol. I., p. 175.

† An Essay towards a Theory of Apparitions, London, 1813, p. 28.

hundred years ago to discover how common were the supposed miraculous events by which whole communities were deceived.* And we see at the present day by the yearly example afforded by the pretended liquefaction of the blood of St. Januarius in Naples, just referred to, that even our own time is not exempt from instances (besides those which illustrate the power of spiritualism in this respect) of large numbers of people being simultaneously subjected to illusions or hallucinations. Thus Hibbert, † quoting from Ellis's edition of Brand's Popular Antiquities, relates the story of a sea captain of Newcastle-upon-Tyne, as follows: "His cook," he said, "chanced to die on their passage homeward. This honest fellow having had one of his legs a little shorter than the other, used to walk in that way which our vulgar idiom calls 'an up and a down.' A few nights after his body had been committed to the deep, our captain was alarmed by his mate with an account that the cook was walking before the ship, and that all hands were on deck to see him. The captain, after an oath or two for having been disturbed, ordered them to let him alone and try which, the ship or he, should first get to Newcastle. But turning out on further importunity, he honestly confessed that he had like to have caught the contagion, for, on seeing something move in a way so similar to that which his old friend used, and withal having a cap on so like that which he was wont to wear, he verily thought there was more in the report than he was at first willing to believe. A general panic diffused itself. He

* For instance "Prodigiorum ac ostentorum Chronicon per Conradum Lycosthenem. Basileæ, MDLVII."

† Sketches of the Philosophy of Apparitions, etc., 2nd edition, Edinburgh, 1825, p. 16.

ordered the ship to be steered towards the object, but not a man would move the helm! Compelled to do this himself, he found on a nearer approach that the ridiculous cause of all their terror was part of a main-top, the remains of some wreck, floating before them. Unless he had ventured to make this nearer approach to the supposed ghost, the tale of the walking cook had long been in the mouths and excited the fears of many honest and very brave fellows in the Wapping of Newcastle-upon-Tyne."

Dr. D. H. Tuke,* in his recent very interesting work, gives the following instance:—

"A curious illustration of the influence of the imagination in magnifying the perceptions of sensorial impressions derived from the outer world, occurred during the conflagration at the Crystal Palace in the winter of 1866-7. When the animals were destroyed by the fire, it was supposed that the chimpanzee had succeeded in escaping from his cage. Attracted to the roof with this expectation in full force, men saw the unhappy animal holding on to it and writhing in agony to get astride one of the iron ribs. It need not be said that its struggles were watched by those below with breathless suspense, and as the newspapers informed us, with 'sickening dread.' But there was no animal whatever there, and all this feeling was thrown away upon a tattered piece of blind, so torn as to resemble to the eye of fancy, the body, arms and legs of an ape."

It is even possible for considerable bodies of men to be affected simultaneously by the same dream. Laurent † relates the following remarkable event:—

* Illustrations of the Influence of the Mind upon the Body in Health and Disease, etc., London, 1872, p. 44.

† Grand Dictionnaire de Médecine, t. xxxiv., Art. Incubi, par M. Parent.

"The first battalion of the regiment of Latour d'Auvergne, of which I was surgeon-major, while in garrison at Palmi in Calabria, received orders to march at once to Tropea in order to oppose the landing from a fleet which threatened that part of the country. It was in the month of June, and the troops had to march about fifty miles. They started at midnight, and did not arrive at their destination till seven o'clock in the evening, resting but little on the way and suffering much from the heat of the sun. When they reached Tropea they found their camp ready and their quarters prepared, but as the battalion had come from the farthest point and was the last to arrive, they were assigned the worst barracks, and thus eight hundred men were lodged in a place which, in ordinary times, would not have sufficed for half their number. They were crowded together on straw placed on the bare ground, and being without covering, were not able to undress. The building in which they were placed was an old, abandoned abbey, and the inhabitants had predicted that they would not be able to stay there all night in peace, as it was frequented by ghosts, which had disturbed other regiments quartered there. We laughed at their credulity; but what was our surprise to hear about midnight the most frightful cries proceeding from every corner of the abbey, and to see the soldiers rushing terrified from the building. I questioned them in regard to the cause of their alarm, and all replied that the devil lived in the building, and that they had seen him enter by an opening, into their room, under the figure of a very large dog with long, black hair, and throwing himself upon their chests for an instant, had disappeared through another opening in the opposite side of the apartment We laughed at their consternation, and endeavored to prove to them that the phenomenon was due to a very simple and natural cause and was only the effect of their imagination; but we failed to convince them, nor could we persuade them to return to their barracks. They passed the night scattered along the sea shore, and in various parts of the town. In the morning I questioned anew the non-commissioned officers and some of the oldest soldiers. They assured me that they were not accessible to fear; that they did not believe in dreams or ghosts, but that they were fully persuaded they had not been deceived as to the reality of the events of the preceding night. They said that they had not fallen asleep when the dog appeared, that they had obtained a good view of him, and that they were almost suffocated when he leaped on their breasts.

"We remained all day at Tropea, and the town being full of troops we were forced to retain the same barracks, but we could not make the soldiers sleep in them again without our promise that we would pass the night with them. I went there at half-past eleven with the commanding officer; the other officers were, more for curiosity's sake than anything else, distributed in the several rooms. We scarcely expected to witness a repetition of the events of the preceding night, for the soldiers had gone to sleep, reassured by the presence of their officers, who remained awake. But about one o'clock, in all the rooms at the same time, the cries of the previous night were repeated, and again the soldiers rushed out to escape the suffocating embraces of the big, black dog. We had all remained awake watching eagerly for what might happen, but, as may be supposed, we had seen nothing.

"The enemy's fleet having disappeared, we returned next day

to Palmi. Since that event we have marched through the kingdom of Naples in all directions, and in all seasons, but the phenomena have not been reproduced. We are of opinion that the forced march which the troops had been obliged to make during a very hot day, by fatiguing the organs of respiration, had weakened the men, and consequently disposed them to experience these attacks of nightmare. The constrained position in which they had been obliged to lie, the fact of their not being undressed, and the bad air they were obliged to breathe, doubtless aided in the production."

There are two forces resulting from vitality, which may or may not be correlative, but which are of such a nature that some of their more unusual manifestations excite the astonishment of the vulgar, and are inexplicable to many who consider themselves learned. These are the mind, and animal electricity. The latter, thanks to the investigations of Nobili, Matteucci, Müller, Du Bois-Reymond, and others, is beginning to be understood, and its phenomena reduced to fixed laws. All our knowledge of animal electricity tends to show that it does not differ in any essential particular from the galvanism developed outside of the body by chemical action; and that the tissues of the organism, the bones, muscles, nerves, etc., act toward it precisely as they do toward the galvanism which passes along an iron or copper wire and sets a telegraphic instrument in operation. It is impossible for us, therefore, to attribute any of the real or false manifestations of modern spiritualism to this force; and those persons who do so, show themselves to be not fully acquainted either with what is asserted of spiritualism, or with electricity in its internal or external relations with the animal body. The idea that tables are moved, knocks made, and apparitions produced by the electricity of the body, is simply absurd.

The mind—under which term are included perception, the intellect, the emotions, and the will—is ordinarily supposed to have its seat wholly in the brain. That its higher manifestations are due to cerebral action is doubtless true; but holding the view that where there is gray nerve-tissue, there nervous power is generated, the writer believes—and physiology and pathology fully support the opinion—that the spinal cord and sympathetic system are capable of originating certain kinds of mental influence, which, when the brain is quiescent, may be wonderfully intensified. The physiology of the nervous system is by no means even tolerably well understood. Science has, for ages, been fettered by theological and metaphysical dogmas, which give the mind an existence independent of the nervous system, and which teach that it is an entity which sets all the functions of the body in action, and of which the brain is the seat. There can be no scientific inquiry relative to matters of faith—facts alone admit of investigation; and hence, so long as psychology was expounded by teachers who had never even seen a human brain, much less a spinal cord or sympathetic nerve, who knew absolutely nothing of nervous physiology, and who, therefore, taught from a stand-point which had not a single fact to rest upon, it was not to be expected that the true science of mind could make much progress. It is different now, but the majority of physiologists have scarcely yet thrown off the trammels of the past, and, therefore, barely going a step in advance of Descartes—who confounded the mind with the soul, and lodged it in the pineal gland—they attribute all mental action to the brain alone.

Before we can be qualified to inquire into the powers of the mind, we must have a definite conception of what mind is. To express the idea in sufficiently full, but yet concise, language is difficult, and perhaps no definition can be given which will be entirely free from objection. For the purposes, however, of the present memoir, the mind may be regarded as a force, the result of nervous action and the elements of which are perception, intellect, the emotions and the will. Of these qualities some reside exclusively in the brain, but the others, as is clearly shown by observation and experiment, cannot be restricted to this organ, but are developed with more or less intensity by other parts of the nervous system. It would be out of place to enter fully into the consideration of the important questions thus touched upon, but in the fact that the spinal cord and sympathetic ganglia are not devoid of mental power we find an explanation of some of the most striking phenomena of what is called spiritualism. To these the attention of the reader will presently be invited.

CHAPTER II.

MAGNETISM IN ITS RELATIONS TO SPIRITUALISM.

IT has been supposed that MAGNETISM—a force correlative with electricity—resides in the body, and that some persons are peculiarly sensitive to the influence of the magnet and to the magnetism evolved by other individuals. This subject has been thoroughly investigated by the Baron von Reichenbach, a very learned, but certainly a very imaginative man, who has developed from his inquiries some truth and a great deal of fancy. He sought to give an explanation of mesmerism, and really succeeded to a certain extent. The following observation is certainly true:

"If a strong magnet, capable of supporting about ten pounds, be drawn downward over the bodies of fifteen or twenty persons, without actually touching them, some among them will always be found to be excited by it in a peculiar manner. The number of people who are sensitive in this way is greater than is generally imagined. . . . The kind of impression produced on these excitable people, who otherwise may be regarded as in perfect health, is scarcely describable; it is rather disagreeable than pleasant, and combined with a slight sensation of cold or warmth, resembling a cool or gently warm breath of air, which the patients imagine to blow softly.

Sometimes they feel sensations of drawing, pricking, or creeping; some complain of sudden attacks of headache. Not only women, but men in the very prime of life, are found distinctly susceptible to this influence; in children it is sometimes very active." *

Reichenbach supposed that these and other phenomena were due to a hitherto undescribed force which he denominated *od*, the *odic force*, or *odyle*, and which was present in the body. When evolved in large quantity, the subjects were said to be sensitive, and could then not only experience the sensations mentioned, but could also see the luminous flames which were asserted to be given off from the poles of a magnet. At first his experiments were conducted with confessedly sickly persons; but he subsequently ascertained that individuals in perfect health were capable of experiencing the same sensations. What the baron's "perfect health" was, will be apparent from the following remarks which conclude his detailed description of thirty-five persons who were thus doubly gifted:

"None of these perfectly healthy persons knew anything about their most remarkable and interesting peculiarities; and they were not a little astonished at the discovery, under my guidance, of powers of which they had never before dreamed. The manner in which I come upon the trace of them, which I at once take up and follow, is now simply this: I inquire among my acquaintance whether they know any one who is frequently troubled with periodical headaches, especially megrim, who complains of temporary oppression of the stomach, or who often sleeps badly without apparent cause, talks in the sleep,

* Physico-Physiological Researches on the Dynamics of Magnetism, etc p. 3. English translation, by Dr. John Ashburner. London, 1851.

rises up or even gets out of bed, or is restless at night during the period of full moon, or to whom the moonlight in general is disagreeable, or who is readily disordered in churches or theatres, or very sensitive to strong smells, grating or shrill noises, etc.,—all such persons, who may be otherwise healthy, I seek after, and make a pass with a finger over the palm of their hands, and scarcely ever miss finding them sensitive. When they follow me into the obscurity of my dark chamber and remain there an hour or two, their surprise is excited by the appearance of a quantity of luminous appearances, of which they had not previously the slightest idea. The number of persons who are in this state of excitability does actually exceed belief, and I state it rather below than above the reality when I say that at least a third part of the population are sensitive; for on every side on which I turn I meet with healthy sensitives; and I could in a few days collect, not dozens, but hundreds, if it were requisite. It will and must soon be proved how little ground there is to doubt these asseverations. Sensitiveness is not a rarity among human beings, as I myself thought some years ago, but a very generally distributed quality, which, after my accounts, will soon be discovered in every direction, and will throw open a new and not unimportant page of the human condition."

Can any physician conversant with the abnormal conditions of the nervous system doubt that such "healthy persons" as those described by the Baron von Reichenbach could be made under "guidance," to see or feel almost any thing suggested to them? The writer has now under his professional care a young lady, hysterical, a somnambulist, and affected with chorea, upon whom this principle of suggestion can be made to act with striking effect, and who would be a perfect godsend to all mesmerizers, mediums, and electro-biologists. For instance, it is only necessary to tell her that certain images are before her, when she directly sees them exactly as they are described; to inform her that she is about to have galvanism applied, and then to give her the unconnected poles, when she at once experiences the shock; to ask her if she has not a bitter or a sweet or a sour taste in her mouth, when she immediately declares that she has just such a taste as is mentioned. Voices are heard and odors smelt precisely as they are described to her. Hundreds of patients affected with diseases of the nervous system are susceptible, in a greater or less degree to the operation of suggestion; and to the action of this principle many miracles and impostures owe the success with which they have been received. To it many of the phenomena of spiritualism are clearly due.

In the *Comptes Rendus* for August 31st, 1874, is a letter from M. Volpicelli, of Rome, to M. Chevreul, which illustrates the effect of the imagination in giving rise to *expected* phenomena. "A physician," says the writer, "possessing an excellent reputation, asserts that if a magnet is brought into contact with a nervous subject the magnetism produces many disquieting effects and notably deranges his health. For my part I do not think these disturbances are in any way due to the magnetic influence, whose real existence, however, I do not contest, but I attribute them to the influence of the person's imagination. I was invited by the learned medical professor to experiment upon a nervous subject at the Hospital Saint Esprit, at Rome. I accepted the courteous offer, but instead of a magnet I brought a piece of iron, which was not in the least magnetized. The patient had no sooner seen this iron than he was seized with violent convulsions; his imagination was so excited that we could observe the greatest intensity of nervous disturbance.

"I made a second experiment: A magnet was placed in the hand of a person likewise affected with a nervous malady; at the end of a few seconds he became so violently excited that I was obliged to remove it. I was impressed with the conviction that the nervous disturbance was produced by the mere sight of the loadstone, and not by any magnetic action, and several days afterward I was able to convince myself by means of the following process: The same person was called upon to preside at a scientific reunion. I took powerful magnets and placed them in his chair, in his table drawer, and even beneath his feet, without his having the slightest suspicion of any of my preparations. During the *séance*, which continued more than two hours, he had no nervous disturbance whatever, and at the conclusion of the meeting he declared, on my asking him, that he felt perfectly well. On being told that he had been surrounded by powerful magnets, he manifested both surprise and fear, as though he were not quite sure of being in perfect health."

But notwithstanding the fact that many of the experiments of the Baron von Reichenbach and others have no other foundation than that property of the human mind which causes it to be subjectively affected by suggestion, it is undoubtedly true that there is a germ of fact in his investigations, and that magnetism is destined to play an important part in physiology and pathology. In a strikingly original and interesting paper*

* "On the Physiological Action of Magnetism." By John Vansant, M.D., etc., Journal of Psychological Medicine, April, 1870.

recently published, the experiments detailed in which have been verified by the writer, it is clearly shown that certain very obvious symptoms are induced by the application of a magnet directly to the body, and that the lower animals and even plants are indubitably affected by its influence.

Nevertheless, there is no proof that magnetism, or the odic force, is capable under any circumstances of producing the clairvoyant state, of moving tables, of causing raps, or that any of the other more striking phenomena that are claimed for spiritualism can be accounted for through its agency. The *possibility* of such a power being exercised is quite another thing. The force that can cause a mass of iron to be moved in opposition to the laws of gravity, and through media impervious to all ordinary influences, can scarcely have the word *impossible* properly applied to it. But this is not a question of possibilities, but of facts, and certainly it has not been shown, with that reasonable degree of certainty which all scientific questions demand, that magnetism in or out of the body exercises any such control over mind or matter as has been claimed by its partisans.

In this connection, and as showing how greatly, sincere and conscientious individuals may be deceived, it may be well to recall the chief points in the history of Angélique Cottin, the "electric girl," who, nearly thirty years ago, created much excitement in France.

According to the account given by Figuier * in his *Histoire du Merveilleux*, this young girl, at this time about fourteen years old, on the fifteenth of January, 1846, was occupied with

* Histoire du Merveilleux dans le Temps Moderne, par Louis Figuier. Deuxième édition. Paris, 1861. t. iv., p. 160.

three companions in her ordinary work, which consisted in weaving silk gloves. It was eight o'clock in the evening, when the oaken round table at which one was seated, suddenly, without obvious cause, became violently agitated, and could not be maintained in its proper position. Frightened at this remark able occurrence, the girls ran away uttering cries of terror and attracting several of the neighbors to the place. Not being able otherwise to convince the spectators of the truth of their story, two of the girls seated themselves again at the table, which, however, remained perfectly still, but the instant Angélique took her place at it, the table was again shaken and finally was completely overturned. At the same time the young girl was apparently compelled to follow the table, but if she touched it another series of violent movements ensued. The conclusion arrived at by the neighbors was that Angélique Cottin was bewitched.

The following day she endeavored to resume her work, but similar results followed. Various plans were devised for keeping the table quiet but all were in vain. Being unable to explain the unusual phenomena otherwise, the people of the village were unanimously of the opinion that Angélique Cottin was possessed by the devil, and accordingly she was taken to the priest to have the fiend exorcised.

But the good father was not disposed to employ the therapeutics of the church unless he were first an eye witness of the satanic manifestations. Accordingly the table was brought, and on Angélique sitting down at it, it was shaken but not overturned. Her own chair was, however, drawn away from the table, and oscillated so violently that she could with difficulty keep her seat.

Convinced of the reality of the phenomena, the priest was still unwilling to employ exorcism for what he regarded as a physical disease requiring medical treatment. He therefore quieted the excitement of the inhabitants by declaring that Angélique was affected with a rare and perhaps unknown disorder, for which physicians should be consulted.

The manifestations continued and became much more varied in character. Books, brushes and other objects were repelled from her if even her clothes touched them. A chair upon which she was about to seat herself was forcibly repulsed, notwithstanding the efforts made by three strong men to keep it in place. Work was no longer possible, for everything she touched was immediately drawn or pushed away with great energy.

Several physicians examined her and were witnesses of the occurrences. The opinion generally entertained was that Angélique was highly charged with electricity, and many experiments undertaken by the doctors and other learned men went to show that this really was the case. Among others, Dr. Lemonier examined into the matter and testified as follows, in a letter which he wrote at the time :

" I hasten to give my views relative to the phenomena which you have observed in the girl Cottin ; they are perfectly well known to me. *I have seen a willow basket filled with beans instantly emptied and the contents scattered round the room, when the young girl placed her left hand in it.* All the furniture, tables, chairs, chests, when touched by her hand were repulsed violently. The procureur du loi of Mortagne was present ; he being seated on a chair, requested Angelique to sit down on his knees. Instantly, as by a thunderbolt, he was raised up and repelled with the chair. Another chair held by myself and two of my friends escaped from our hands, and *one of the legs of this chair was broken.* The girl uttered a cry indicative of pain when any one put any thing in her hand. Placed on a chair isolated from the ground by four glasses, the girl supporting her feet on the rung, produced no manifestations. But as soon as she was placed in contact with the floor the phenomena recommenced, and always from left to right. During a paroxysm one side was warmer than the other. Moreover there was an unusual excitement of the circulation."

There were many other similar letters, and Dr. Tauchon wrote a *brochure* entitled: *Enquiry relative to the reality of the electrical phenomena of Angélique Cottin,** in which the manifestations are very fully described and many arguments adduced in favor of their reality.

But in an evil moment for the continuance of the remarkable phenomena exhibited in the person of Angelique, her parents, prompted by a desire to turn an honest penny by making a show of their daughter, resolved to travel with her from city to city, and eventually to take her to Paris. The manifestations continued, many other physicians and scientific men examined her, and were satisfied that no more was claimed for her than was actually founded on fact. Finally she arrived in Paris, and a commission of the Academy of Sciences, composed of Arago, Becquerel, Isidore Geoffroy, Saint Hilaire, Bobriest, Rayer and Pariset, was appointed to examine her and report the facts to the Academy. The inquiry was entered into with calmness and deliberation, instruments were

* Enquête sur l'Authenticité des Phenomènes Electriques d'Angélique Cottin. G. Baillière, Paris, 1846.

employed to determine the quantity of electricity evolved by the "electric girl," and the following report was made:—

"We were assured that M'lle Cottin exercised a strong, repulsive action over bodies of every kind at the instant that any part of her clothing touched them. It was also said that tables were overturned by touching them with a single thread of silk held in her hand.

"No appreciable effect of this kind was produced before the commission.

"In the accounts communicated to the Academy, it was alleged that a magnetic needle, influenced by the arm of the young girl, at first rapidly oscillated and then assumed a position far from the magnetic meridian.

"Before the commission, such a needle, delicately suspended, experienced, under such circumstances, neither permanent nor temporary displacement.

"M. Tauchon believes that M'lle Cottin has the faculty of distinguishing the north from the south pole of a magnet by simply touching it with her fingers.

"The commission is convinced, by numerous and varied experiments, that the young girl does not possess this power.

"The commission will not pursue much further the enumeration of its failures. It will only say that the only fact announced which was realized before it was that of sudden and violent movements in chairs on which the young girl was seated. Suspicions having been aroused relative to the manner by which these movements were produced, it was determined to submit them to careful examination. The commission announced, without reserve, that the researches would be directed to the point of ascertaining what part certain quick though concealed movements of the hands and feet might have in the causation of the alleged facts. At this period it was declared to us that the young girl had lost her faculties of attraction and repulsion, and that we would be notified as soon as they were regained. Although several days have elapsed since then, the commission has not received the promised notice, though we have been informed that M'lle Cottin daily repeats her performances before others.

"After having duly weighed all the circumstances, the commission is of the opinion that the allegations made to the Academy relative to M'lle Angélique Cottin should be considered as not proven."

Nothing more was heard of the "electrical girl." Like many other extraordinary occurrences, her performances were incapable of resisting the inquiries of scientific men, not easily led astray by their emotions, but bringing to the investigation a desire to know the truth, and a determination to be guided only by facts.

CHAPTER III.

CONCENTRATED ATTENTION A SOURCE OF ERRONEOUS SENSORIAL IMPRESSIONS.

THE attention, when concentrated upon any particular thing or part of the body, will often lead to erroneous sensorial impressions. An observer gazing anxiously out to sea, or across a vast plain, will scarcely ever fail to see the object of which he is in search; an expectant watcher hears every moment the rumbling of wheels, the footstep, or the knock which announces the wished-for or dreaded arrival; and pains, tastes, odors, and even diseases, can frequently be thus originated. Thus, a lady who has been under the professional care of the writer for intense nervous headaches, and who is of a very impressionable organization, is able at will to produce a pain in any part of her body by steadily fixing her attention upon it. Even the mention in her presence of physical suffering experienced by other persons immediately results in her feeling similar pains to those described, in corresponding parts of her own body. The case of Mrs. A., detailed by Sir David Brewster,* is a forcible illustration of the point in question. This lady, who possessed a remarkable degree of good sense, and who was subject at one time to hallucinations of various kinds, was of so sensitive a nature that the account of a person having suffered pain of any kind, immediately produced corresponding twitches in the same part of her own body. The mention, for instance,

* Letters on Natural Magic addressed to Sir Walter Scott. Letter III.

of the surgical operation of amputating an arm, at once caused her to feel a severe pain in her arm. She talked in her sleep, and was accustomed to exercise her memory greatly by writing verses of poetry—facts which showed the existence of a morbidly hyperæsthetic nervous system rendered still more excitable by the undue development of her imagination.

Physicians know very well that actual organic disease may be produced by the habitual concentration of the attention on an organ. The fancies of the hypochondriac may thus in time become realities.

Many of the facts of spiritualism are clearly explainable by referring them to this influence.

A so-called "spiritual photograph" is shown to a sorrowing mother, and immediately she recognizes the features of her dead son; the wish is in such cases father to the thought. I have repeatedly known the same photograph acknowledged to be the exact likeness of several very different persons, solely because those who looked at it and carefully examined every feature, were told beforehand that it was a correct portrait of some one in whom they were specially interested.

An experiment illustrating how the sense of sight may be perverted by the concentration of the attention, may be readily made by any one. Let him go out into the middle of Union Square, for instance, and look steadily towards the zenith, at nothing.—In a few minutes he will have a crowd about him, all gazing eagerly in the same direction. He need not utter a word, not even in reply to the questions that may be asked him. In a short time some one will declare he sees something, another will see a bird far up in the air, another a star, another a balloon, and so on. Then let the original observer declare the object to be a kite or any other thing which it is possible to see in the sky, and forthwith many present will at once agree that it is a kite, while all the time their sense of vision is being deceived by an unreal image.

A timid woman goes to bed after having read accounts or listened to stories of house-burnings. Her attention is concentrated upon the one object, and before she goes to sleep she sees lights, hears the crackling of the flames and smells the smoke. I once knew a lady who not only under these circumstances experienced all these sensations mentioned, but who even felt a feeling of suffocation from the smoke which she imagined filled the room.

In his book on Hypnotism to which fuller reference will presently be made, Mr. Braid says that on one occasion he requested four gentlemen to lay their arms on a table with the palms of their hands upwards, each one to look at the palm of his hand for a few minutes, and at the same time concentrating his attention on it and to wait for the result. In about five minutes, the first, one of the present members of the Royal Academy, stated that he felt a sensation of great cold in the hands; another, who is a very talented author, said that for some time he hought nothing was going to happen, but at last a darting picking sensation took place from the palm of the hand, as if electric sparks were being drawn from it; the third gentleman, lately mayor of a large borough, said that he felt a very uncomfortable sensation of heat come over his hand; the fourth, secretary to an important association, had become rigidly cataleptic, his arm being firmly fixed to the table.

I am very sure, with the great John Hunter, that it is impossible for any one to concentrate the attention on any part of the body, without having, as the result, a sensation of some kind originate therein.

It is perfectly within the range of our experience that many who go to witness the performances of mediums should, upon being told to fix the attention on a certain event which was about to take place, experience the sensation through the sight, hearing, touch or smell, that the event did in reality occur, when in fact they have been deceived. Upon one occasion I was present when a medium announced that he was about to increase his height. He disappeared behind a screen, and on emerging to view, every one present, except myself, perceived an increase of height which they variously fixed at from five to eight inches. But I had taken the precaution to measure with my eye the distance from the top of his head to the chandelier under which he stood, and I saw that he almost touched it. When he came from behind the screen and stood under the chandelier it was very evident that the increase in height consisted of about two inches, an amount which any tall man can at will apparently add to his stature.

The visions of saints, votaries and other enthusiasts, about which I shall have more to say under another head, are, in a great measure, the result of concentrated attention upon some one object or image.

CHAPTER IV.

SLEIGHT OF HAND COMPARED TO SPIRITUALISTIC MANIFESTATIONS.

A STILL more important factor in the production of spiritualistic manifestations is sleight of hand. The perfection to which this art is carried by accomplished performers is really remarkable, and is much more wonderful than would be real visitations of spirits. For when we are dealing with what appear to be circumstances and conditions of every-day life and are deceived, with all the elements of knowledge at our command, it is certainly more astonishing than would be the actual appearance before our eyes of something which no one had ever seen before and of which no one knew anything.

For instance, a man stands before us clothed in ordinary apparel, and on an open stage of a theatre, with no drapery within reach, and nothing to obstruct our full view of him. He takes a white cambric handkerchief out of his coat pocket, and holds it in both hands stretched out before him. He then, still holding one corner with his left hand, seizes the other corner with his teeth and with the free right hand proceeds to take from under the handkerchief bowl after bowl, to the number of a dozen, full of water to the brim and each containing several gold fish. Another places a stool in full view of the spectators, and on this stool puts a large empty basket. There is no curtain around the stool, and it would apparently be impossible for anything to pass through the bottom of the basket without being seen by every one present. A woman then gets into the basket, the lid is closed, and the performer, drawing a long sharp sword, plunges it in all directions into the basket. Shrieks and groans, gradually getting fainter and fainter, apparently come from the basket; blood, or what has the appearance of blood, drops from the sword, and finally, the cries having ceased, the performer desists from his horribly realistic performance, during which several ladies have fainted, and announces that he has done a part of his task, and will now proceed to its conclusion. He calls loudly in an unknown tongue, and straightway the woman who had entered the basket walks into the room from the farther end, and takes her place upon the stage with as much *sang-froid* as though she had not been just butchered in presence of four or five hundred people.

Now, such things are to me more wonderful, deceptions as they are avowed to be, than would be the apparition of a ghost of a person I knew to be dead. A man in evening dress can not reasonably be supposed to be able to carry a dozen gallon bowls full of water and fish in his waistcoat pockets. Such capacity is not for a moment to be admitted, and yet he in some way or other deceives the eyes of the hundreds of persons who are watching him with every intention of detecting him if they can. A woman enters an empty basket and gets out in full presence of many people without any one seeing her leave, while the attention of all is concentrated upon the place where she is. If the spirit of Julius Cæsar should appear to me I should not be as much confounded as by this performance. I know nothing of Julius Cæsar's spirit, of its attributes, or of the circumstances of its visibility or invisibility, I do not even know that it exists. I neither believe or disbelieve in its existence. That of which nothing is known, cannot excite astonishment, for we are only astonished when our preconceived notions of things are suddenly overturned. But the conviction of a woman going into a basket is, that she cannot get out of it, in our pressence and within our view, without our knowledge, and when she does get out under these circumstances we are naturally astonished.

A sleight of hand performer knows very well the great advantage of being able to engage the attention of those whom he is deceiving. Mention has already been made of this element as a source of inattention to other things which are going on around. The fact that individuals have been severely wounded in battle without knowing it till faintness supervened, or the contest was over, is a familiar fact, but it is not so generally known that surgical operations requiring much time for their successful performance and causing great pain under ordinary circumstances, can be effected without the patient experiencing the least suffering simply by engaging the attention in such a way as to produce a kind of mental exaltation. It was undoubtedly this emotional excitement which prevented sensation in those who in former times were put to torture or burnt at the stake for their opinions.

When, in addition, the performer is enabled to accompany his operations with imposing rites and ceremonies or an appearance of mystery or awe, his success with a certain class of observers is still more certain, for not only does he deceive their senses but he imposes on their understandings.

This was the case in the incantations used to convince

Benvenuto Cellini, and as the story is exceedingly apposite in the present connection, I quote it as told by himself. *

"It happened through a variety of odd accidents, that I made acquaintance with a Sicilian priest, who was a man of genius and well versed in the Latin and Greek authors. Happening one day to have some conversation with him on the art of necromancy, I, who had a great desire to know something of the matter, told him that I had all my life felt a curiosity to be acquainted with the mysteries of this art. The priest made answer 'that the man must be of a resolute and strong temper who enters upon that study.' I replied 'that I had fortitude and ambition enough if I could but find an opportunity.' The priest subjoined: 'If you think you have the heart to venture, I will give you all the satisfaction you can desire.' Thus we agreed to undertake this matter.

"The priest, one evening, prepared to satisfy me, and desired me to look out for a companion or two. I invited one Vincenzio Romoli, who was my intimate acquaintance. He brought with him a native of Pistoria, who cultivated the black art himself. We repaired to the Colosseo, and the priest, according to the custom of necromancers, began to draw circles upon the ground with the most impressive ceremonies imaginable; he likewise brought thither, assafoetida, several precious perfumes, and fire, with some combustions, which diffused noxious odors. As soon as he was in readiness, he made an opening in the circle, and, having taken us by the hand, ordered the other necromancer, his partner, to throw the perfume into the fire at the proper time, intrusting the care of the

* Memoirs of Benvenuto Cellini, written by himself. Roscoe's Translation: London, 1823, Vol. i., p. 236.

fire and the perfumes to the rest, and then he began his incantations. This ceremony lasted above an hour and a half, when there appeared several legions of devils, inasmuch, that the amphitheatre was quite filled with them.

I was busy about the perfumes, when the priest, perceiving there was a considerable number of infernal spirits, turned to me and said: 'Benvenuto, ask them something.' I answered, Let them bring me into the company of my Sicilian mistress, Angelica.' That night we obtained no answer of any sort; but I have received great satisfaction in having my curiosity so far indulged. The necromancer told me it was requisite we should go a second time, assuring me that I should be satisfied in whatever I asked, but that I must bring with me a pure and immaculate boy.

"I took with me a youth, who was in my service, of about twelve years of age, together with the same Vincenzio Romoli, who had been my companion the first time, and one Agnolino Gaddi, an intimate acquaintance, whom I likewise prevailed upon to assist at the ceremony. When we came to the place appointed, the priest, having made his preparations as before, with the same, and even more startling ceremonies, placed us within the circle which he had likewise drawn, with a more wonderful art and in a more solemn manner than at our former meeting. Then, having committed the care of the perfumes and the fire to my friend, Vincenzio, who was assisted by Agnolino Gaddi, he put into my hands a pintaculo or magical chart, and bid me turn it towards the places that he should direct me, and under the pintaculo I held my boy. The necromancer, having began to make his tremendous invocations, called by their names, a multitude of demons, who were the leaders of the several legions, and invoked the virtue and power of the eternal and uncreated God who lives forever, in the Hebrew language as likewise in Latin and Greek; inasmuch that the amphitheatre was almost in an instant filled with demons, a hundred times more numerous than at the former conjuration. Vincenzio Romoli was busied in making a fire, with the assistance of Agnolino, and burning a great quantity of precious perfumes. I, by the direction of the necromancer, again desired to be in the company of my Angelica. The former, thereupon, turning to me, said, 'know they have declared that in the space of a month, you shall be in her company.'

"He then requested me to stand resolutely by him because the legions were now above a thousand more in number than he had designed, and besides these were the most dangerous, so that after they had answered my question, it behooved him to be civil to them and dismiss them quietly. At the same time the boy under the pintaculo was in a terrible fright, saying that there were in that place a million of fierce men who threatened to destroy us, and that moreover four armed giants of an enormous stature were endeavoring to break into our circle. During this time, whilst the necromancer, trembling with fear, endeavored by mild and gentle methods to dismiss them in the best way he could, Vincenzio Romoli, who quivered like an aspen leaf, took care of the perfumes. Though I was as much terrified as any of them, I did my utmost to conceal the terror I felt, so that I greatly contributed to inspire the rest with resolution; but the truth is I gave myself over for a dead man. Seeing the horrid fright the necromancer was in, the boy placed his head between his knees and said: 'In this posture will I die for we shall all surely perish.' I told him that all these demons were under us, and what he saw was smoke and shadow, so bid him hold up his head and take courage. No sooner did he look up but he cried out, 'the whole amphitheatre is burning and the fire is just falling upon us,' so covering his eyes with his hands, he again exclaimed that destruction was inevitable and he desired to see no more. The necromancer entreated me to have a good heart and take care to burn proper perfumes; upon which I turned to Romoli and bid him burn all the most precious perfumes he had. At the same time I cast my eyes upon Agnolino Taddi, who was terrified to such a degree that he could scarce distinguish objects, and seemed to be half dead. Seeing him in this condition, I said, 'Agnolino, upon these occasions a man should not yield to fear, but should stir about and give his assistance; so come directly and put on some more of these perfumes.' Poor Agnolino, upon attempting to move, was so violently terrified that the effects of his fear overpowered all the perfumes we were burning. The boy hearing a crepitation, ventured once more to raise his head, when seeing me laugh, he began to take courage, and said that the devils were flying away with a vengeance.

"In this condition we stayed till the bell rang for morning prayer. The boy again told us that there remained but few devils, and these were at a great distance. When the magician had performed the rest of his ceremonies, he stripped off his gown and took up a wallet full of books which he had brought with him. We all went out of the circle together, keeping as close to each other as we possibly could, especially the boy, who had placed himself in the middle holding the necromancer by the coat and me by the cloak. As we were going to our houses in the quarter of Banchi, the boy told us that two of the demons whom we had seen at the amphitheatre went on before us, leaping and skipping, sometimes running upon the roofs of the houses, and sometimes upon the ground."

As Cellini was constantly the subject of hallucinations, he was a fit person to be imposed upon by the priest, who, as Roscoe states in a note, probably made use of the magic lantern to throw images of demons on the clouds of smoke raised by the wood and perfumes. It will be noticed that the only one who saw the demons where there was no smoke, was the boy, who was evidently in such a condition of terror and excitement as not to be very clear in his perception. Cellini naively adds that all dreamed that night of nothing but devils.

Subsequently, as the time approached for the fulfilment of the promise, and as Cellini became anxious, the priest knowing that he could not bring Angelica to Rome, contrived a plan for sending Cellini to Naples, and thus apparently showing the good faith of the demons and his own power. He fastened a quarrel on him, and then making Cellini believe that he had killed his adversary, persuaded him through emissaries to flee from Rome in order to save himself from the wrath of the Pope. Cellini went to Naples, and was in the company of his Angelica within the month.

Many instances have come to my knowledge in which similar conduct by mediums of the present day, has equally led to the deceptions of their dupes.

In one case, a lady consulted a well-known orthodox medium, relative to the opinion of her deceased mother, in the matter of her marriage to a young man of rather questionable position and character. Knowing that the lady intended to visit the medium, the lover went first and fully posted the necromancer in many of the details of the mother's life, and expressed his own strong desire, liberally supported by greenback arguments, that the advice should be in favor of the marriage. The young lady went; the mother appeared; the questions were answered, most unequivocally in favor of the mar riage, and the lover was extolled as a model of goodness and propriety. The recarnified spirit was clothed in white, and the lady noticed that the gown worn was marked with her mother's name. She retired perfectly satisfied, and immediately announced her engagement. But the accepted lover saw fit, soon afterwards, to change his mind, and his reputation being already bad, he thought it better to have the engagement broken by the lady rather than himself. He therefore caused the medium to write a series of letters to the lady in her mother's name, in which it was stated, that, since the first communication, circumstances had come to light, which were not then known, and that, therefore, having her daughter's happiness at heart, she felt bound to urge her daughter not to marry the man to whom she was engaged. These letters were signed exactly as her mother wrote her name. The daughter, who, it must be confessed, was a fit subject for mediumistic wiles, at once broke off the engagement, and the young man had the effrontery to tell her how he had contrived the whole business, even to furnishing the medium with a night gown, belonging to the deceased mother, and marked with her name.

Elephas Levi,* in his chapters on necromancy, gives very elaborate directions for raising the dead. Thus, the operator is to go every evening at the same hour, into a dimly lighted cham

* Dogme et rituel de la haute magie, t. II, Paris, 1861, p. 18.

ber, a room in which the dead person was accustomed to sit, and then placing the single lamp behind him, is to gaze fixedly, and in silence, at the portrait of the deceased. The room is then to be perfumed with good incense, and the necromancer is to retire backwards.

On the day fixed for the evocation, the one who proposes to raise the dead, should dress himself as for a *fête;* should not begin a conversation with any one, and he should eat only a single meal of bread, wine and roots or fruits. The table-cloth must be immaculately white, two covers are to be laid for two persons, a piece of bread placed at the plate representing the dead person, and a few drops of wine in the wine-glass. The meal is to be eaten in silence in the chamber of evocation, and before the portrait of the person to be recalled to earth. Then the remains of the repast are to be removed with the exception of the bread and wine, which are to be left standing before the portrait.

In the evening at the hour of the deceased's habitual visit, the chamber should be entered in silence. A fire is to be lighted with cypress wood, and into it incense is to be thrown at the same time that the name of the dead person is pronounced. The fire and the lamp are then to be allowed to die out. This day the veil is not to be removed from the portrait.

When the flame of the fire has ceased, incense is to be thrown on the embers, and God is to be invoked according to the formulas of the religion which the deceased professed, and according to the ideas which he entertained of God.

In making this prayer it is necessary for the evoker to identify himself with the person to be evoked, to speak as he spoke, and in a measure to believe himself to be the person whose presence is desired. Then after a quarter of an hour of silence to speak to him as if he were present, with affection and with faith praying him to appear. Then cover the face with both hands and renew this prayer, and then in a loud voice call the person by name three times. Falling on the knees, the eyes closed or covered, and speaking to him mentally, the advent is to be awaited for several minutes, then again call three times in a low and tender voice, and slowly open the eyes. If nothing is seen, repeat the experiment the following year, and a third time if necessary. It is certain that at farthest on the third occasion the dead person will appear, and the longer the appearance is delayed the more real and visible it will be.

Nervous and impressionable people would, as most physicians know, be very apt to be so impressed by such stuff as this as to experience the hallucination of seeing the person called upon. For the purpose, the formula is a good one, and its use by some people who have come under my observation, would scarcely fail to bring the dead visibly before their eyes.

That some of the phenomena of spiritualism are explainable on the theory that they result from sleight of hand, and natural magic, is not to be doubted. The perfection to which such performances can be brought is remarkable; and in the East Indies the jugglers far surpass in dexterity any mediums yet produced in the Western world, and they do not pretend that their performances are anything more than adroit tricks. Thus the Hindoo magician causes flowers to grow several feet in a few minutes, changes his rod into a serpent, suspends himself in the air, kills people and restores them to life, and even allows himself to be buried several months in the earth to be dug up at the end of that time alive.

A short time since I invited several medical and other friends to witness in my library some surprising spiritualistic exhibitions by a first class "medium." The operator went through all the performances of the Davenport brothers to the entire satisfaction of the audience. He was securely tied by a gentleman who had been an officer in the naval service and who exhausted his strength and ingenuity in devising bands and knots. A screen was then placed in front of the "medium" and in an instant an accordeon was played, a bell rung and a tambourine struck. The performer then requested that the screen might be removed, and on this being done, he was found to be tied in precisely the same manner as at first. The gentleman who had bound him declared that not a cord or a knot had been interfered with. In a second attempt, the "medium," tied with additional care, rang a bell and was discovered intact in a second afterward.

The rapping of this gentleman was perfect, and he read communications from the dead, made on plain slips of paper, with a skill equal to that of the most highly gifted and orthodox medium.

The astonishment of the audience was great when he informed them that all his performances were deceptions, which he then proceeded to explain in the most satisfactory manner.

But even the doings of this gentleman are exceeded by those of Messrs. Maskelyne and Cooke, who for several years past have been astonishing large numbers of people in London and other parts of Great Britain. Several years previously Mr. Maskelyne made many visits to the *séances* of the Davenport brothers, and becoming convinced that they were impostors, determined to exceed them in the performance of similar ac s, but with the distinct avowal that these were done by legerdemain, and not by spirits. So perfect are his feats, that spiritualists, notwithstanding his denial, insist upon it that he is aided by spiritual power.

In conjunction with Mr. Cooke, all the most astonishing tricks of the Davenports are exceeded. Thus, while securely tied and sealed by gentlemen from the audience, and with both hands filled with flour, Mr. Maskelyne takes off his coat and vest and throws them out of the cabinet, while the coat of any one who may offer appears suddenly on the back of the conjuror, who, when inspected, is found tied and sealed as at first with his hands still full of flour and not a particle of it on the floor.

Mr. Cooke, while equally securely fastened and subjected to checks, drinks a glass of water, drives nails into wood and cuts devices out of paper with a pair of scissors, and still further bewilders the spectators by extricating himself from his bonds and the meshes of a net in which he is enveloped, without the most searching individual of the audience being able to ascertain how the feats are accomplished.

But the most wonderful feature exhibited by these magicians is an automaton called Psycho. It consists of a figure twenty-two inches high, dressed in an oriental costume and sitting cross-legged on a small pedestal. The small size of the figure entirely precludes the idea of anyone being inside; and besides, it may be opened and inspected as thoroughly as may be wished. It is then seen to be filled with machinery, as is also the pedestal on which it is seated. Further, in order to show that there is no communication between the figure and any outside influence it is placed upon an empty cylinder of transparent glass, and this may also be inspected. The whole arrangement is then deposited on the floor, entirely clear from all curtains, traps, or other contrivances. Any one from the audience is allowed to examine all the surroundings and to watch as closely as possible while the performances are going on.

Under these circumstances Psycho plays whist, calculates problems in arithmetic, and acts as a conjuror. Any numbers proposed by the audience are added, subtracted, multiplied or divided with entire accuracy. The results are shown, one figure at a time, by the automaton opening a little door and by a movement of the left hand sliding the figure in front of the aperture.

This automaton plays whist and does various tricks with cards, all of which show intelligence somewhere, but the source of this has hitherto escaped detection. Electricity and magnetism have each been supposed to be the agent, but opportunity has been afforded for full investigation, and it has been shown that to neither, can the intellectual or motive power be ascribed. *

But in the way of conjuring, nothing can exceed the skill of the East Indian Jugglers, some of whom have recently been giving the Prince of Wales exhibitions of their powers. Two hundred and fifty years ago, if we may believe the accounts which have come down to us, they were even more expert than now.

* For a fuller account of Messrs. Maskelyne and Cooke's exploits the reader is referred to a work from which these particulars have been taken, Frost's "Lives of the Conjurors" London, 1876.

Thus, Sir Thomas Roe, who visited India in 1615, charged with a mission from the East India Company to the Emperor Jehangire, saw many magical performances, but his time and attention being otherwise occupied, he gave little heed to such matters. But the Emperor relates that he once witnessed the feats of some Bengalese conjurors and jugglers, the astonishing character of which throws the performances of Mr. Home and all other accomplished "mediums" entirely in the shade.

The conjurors were desired to produce upon the spot, and from seed, ten mulberry trees. They immediately planted ten seeds, which, in a few minutes produced as many trees, each as it grew into the air, spreading forth its branches and yielding excellent fruit. In like manner, apple, fig, almond, walnut and mango trees were produced, all yielding fruit which Jehangire assured us was of the finest quality.

But this was not all, "Before the trees were removed" says the imperial author, "there appeared among the foliage, birds of such surprising beauty in color and shape, and melody of song as the world never saw before. At the close of the operation, the foliage as in autumn, was seen to put on its varied tints, and the trees gradually disappeared into the earth from which they had been made to spring." Major Price stated many years ago that he had himself witnessed similar feats in India, but that a sheet was employed to cover the process. "I have, however," he adds, no "conception of the means by which they were accomplished, unless the jugglers had the trees about them, in every stage, from the seedling to the fruit."

"One night," continues Jehangire, "and in the very middle of the night, when half this globe was wrapped in darkness, one of these seven men stripped himself almost naked, and having spun himself round several times, took a sheet with which he covered himself, and from beneath the sheet drew out a splendid mirror, by the radiance of which, a light so powerful was produced, as to illuminate the hemisphere to an incredible distance around; to such a distance indeed, that we have the attestation of travellers to the fact, who declared that on the night on which the exhibition took place, and at the distance of ten days' journey, they saw the atmosphere so powerfully illuminated as to exceed the brightness of the brightest day they had ever seen.

"They placed in my presence a large cauldron, and partly filling it with water, threw into it eight of the smaller maunds of Irak of rice; when, without the smallest spark of fire, the cauldron began to boil, and in a little time they took off the lid and drew from it nearly a hundred platters full, each with a stewed fowl at the top. They produced a man whom they divided limb from limb, actually severing his head from the body. They scattered these members along the ground, and in this state they laid for some time. They then extended a sheet over the spot, and one of the men went beneath it and in a few minutes came out followed by the individual supposed to have been cut into joints, in perfect health and condition, and one might have easily known that he never received any injury."

This trick was performed in this city about three years ago in the spectacular play called "Roi Carotte," with the addition that the amputated parts were apparently boiled in a cauldron. It was also introduced into London in 1874 by the conjuror Dr. Lynn.

But to return to the Emperor Jehangire and the marvels he witnessed.

"They caused," he says, "two tents to be set up, one at the distance of a bowshot from the other, the entrances being exactly opposite; they raised the canvas all around and desired that it might be particularly observed that the tents were empty. Then fixing them to the ground, two of the men entered, one into each tent. Thus prepared, they said they would undertake to bring out of the tents any animal we chose to mention, whether bird or beast and set them in conflict with each other. Khaun-e-Jahaun, with a smile of incredulity, required them to show us a battle between two ostriches. In a few minutes two ostriches of the largest size issued, one from each tent, and attacked each other with such fury that blood was seen streaming from their heads; they were so equally matched, however, that neither could get the better of the other, and they were therefore separated by the men and conveyed within the tents. They continued to produce from either tent whatever animal we chose to name, and before our eyes set them to fight in the manner I have attempted to describe; and although I have exhausted my utmost invention to discover the secret of the contrivances, it has been entirely without success."

"They were furnished with a bow and about fifty steel pointed arrows. One of the men took the bow and shooting an arrow into the air, the shaft stood fixed at a considerable height; he shot a second arrow which flew straight to the first, to which it became attached, and so with every one of the remaining arrows, to the last of all, which striking the sheaf suspended in the air, the whole immediately broke asunder and came at once to the ground."

"They produced a chain fifty cubits in length, and, in my

presence, threw one end of it towards the sky, where it remained as if fastened to something in the air. A dog was then brought forward, and being placed at the lower end of the chain, immediately ran up it and reaching the other end disappeared in the air. In the same manner a hog, a panther, a lion and a tiger were successively sent up the chain and all disappeared at the upper end. At last they took down the chain and put it into a bag; no one ever discovering in what way the animals were made to vanish into the air in the mysterious manner described."*

The levitation, bodily extension, holding live coals, etc., of Mr. Home are extremely insignificant and sorry performances when compared with those of the jugglers who exhibited before the Emperor Jehangire.

It would be very easy to adduce other instances of legerdemain fully as remarkable as those cited, but the foregoing are sufficient to establish the point that there is nothing claimed by the most deluded believer in spiritualism as being performed by mediums, which is not equalled or excelled by the feats of magicians and jugglers, who do not pretend to be endowed with supernatural powers.

* Lives of the Conjurors, p. 94.

CHAPTER V.

THE DIFFERENT KINDS OF MEDIUMS.

THERE are two classes of mediums, the dishonest and the honest. The former have already engaged a portion of our attention. They are the charlatans who act under false pretences, the Katie Kings, the Davenports, the Fays, and others—whose whole life is one of deceit and fraud—and who charge high prices for very poor exhibitions of jugglery. The others are a peculiar set of individuals, sometimes males, but generally females, who are the subjects of one or more hysteroid affections, engrafted upon a naturally impressionable and irritable nervous organization. Although these people present no essential points of difference, so far as their neurotic dispositions and tendencies are concerned, there are various kinds of mediums as regards capacity and power. According to Allan Kardec,* every person who feels in any way, and to any extent, the influence of the spirits, is a medium. The faculty is one which is inherent in the human race, and is not therefore the peculiar privilege of a few. But some are more highly gifted than others, some exhibit a peculiar aptitude for one or more phenomenal manifestations, and it is to these that the name of medium is commonly applied. Thus, as stated by Kardec, who, under his *nom de plume*, is the leading French authority on spiritualistic science, there are *physical mediums*, such as the table turners, the

* Le livre des médiums, dixième édition. Paris, 1863, p. 195.

fire eaters, levitators, etc.; *sensitive or impressible mediums*, those who have vague impressions, a sort of tingling in the limbs which does not admit of accurate description; *auditive mediums*, who hear spirit voices, which may be either an internal or an external voice; *speaking mediums*, those who exhort and give utterance to communications received from spirits; *seeing mediums*, who are gifted with the faculty of seeing spirits, either when awake or in a state of somnambulism; *somnambulic mediums*, who differ from other kinds in the fact that they act under the influence of their own spirits instead of that of another; *curing mediums*, who are endowed with the power of curing the subjects of various diseases by simply touching them, looking at them, by a gesture, or by addressing a few words to them, without using any medical means whatever; *pneumatographic mediums*, who are able to obtain writing directly from the spirits, a rare gift, as M. Kardec says, and *writing or psychographic mediums*, through whom the spirits communicate their wishes and opinions by causing them to write. To which I would add the *possessed mediums*, those into whose bodies the spirits enter and rend them and contort them, and the *obsessed mediums*, who are seized by the spirits and hurled about from one spot to another. I propose in the following pages to give an explanation of the real conditions which induce each of the kinds of mediumship mentioned by Kardec or myself, and to bring forward examples to show how readily the phenomena are explained upon very different theories than the spiritualistic.

CHAPTER VI.

PHYSICAL MEDIUMS.

A PHYSICAL medium is one who through spiritual agency is able to perform mechanical or chemical feats without the use of mechanical or chemical means, or even to do things which are not from a human point of view regarded as possible with any means or by any power at our command. Increasing the height of the body, suspension of the body in the air, playing on musical instruments, increasing the weights of substances, holding live coals in the hand, etc., are instances of the ability which first class mediums of this kind are claimed to possess. As we have seen, there are many tricks of legerdemain which are fully equal, indeed superior in apparent impossibility, to any one of these things; but I propose to discuss some of these assumed faculties with more particularity than when they were referred to in the chapter on sleight of hand.

Increasing and diminishing the stature. This is one of Mr. Home's favorite performances. The account is given by Mr. Home,* but on the authority of Mr. Jencken, who thus details the occurrence.

"Mr. Home had by this time passed into a trance. After making several circuits and mesmerizing us, he placed himself

* Incidents in my Life, second series. New York, 1872, p. 177.

behind Mrs. ——, whom he mesmerized. I have not space to describe the whole of the proceedings, though I have kept for my own satisfaction accurate notes of what passed. Remarkable was the breathing of Mr. Home on Mrs. ——'s spine, causing alternately a feeling of cold and then of intense heat. Mr. Home said, 'I am now going to grow taller,' and then the remarkable phenomenon of elongation was witnessed. The elongation repeated itself three times. The first time Mr. Home lengthened to about six feet nine inches. And then he shortened down below his normal height to about five feet. He then asked me to hold his feet, which I did by planting my foot on his instep whilst Mr. —— held his head, his left hand being placed on his left shoulder. We carefully measured the extent of elongation against the wall; it showed eight inches. Mr. ——, who had been watching the extension at the waist, measured six inches elongation! Mr. ——, who stood behind Mr. Home barely reached up to his shoulders, though himself six feet high. Mr. Home had now seated himself. Again he said, 'I am going to be elongated (?). Daniel will be elongated thirty times during his life; this is the sixth time.' Mrs. —— who sat next to Mr. Home, placed her hand on his head and her feet on his feet. Thus held, the elongation nevertheless proceeded, measuring six inches. I repeat, Mr. Home was seated all the time and held by those present, anxious to verify this truly unaccountable phenomenon. By this time Mr. Home had awakened from his trance. Shadows on the wall were seen, voices heard, and finally, 'Good-night,' spelt out, terminating the evening."

Upon a previous occasion, according to Mr. Jencken, Mr. Home mesmerized those present, and then telling them what he was going to do, his body was lengthened to almost six feet nine inches.

And again, in presence of Mr. and Mrs. S. C. Hall and a Mr. H. T. Humphreys, who is the reporter, Mr. Home was elongated to the extent of seven feet and contracted to less than five feet.

The fact that upon two of these occasions the spectators were "magnetized" is sufficient to throw the evidence of one of them as regards what took place while he was in that condition entirely beyond the pale of legitimate testimony. The additional fact that at both of these *séances* Mr. Home announced beforehand what he was going to do, brings in the principle of suggestion as a disturbing factor upon individuals avowedly of nervous and highly impressionable temperaments. But in regard to both these occasions, as well as to that at which Mr. and Mrs. S. C. Hall assisted, in which it does not appear that those present were either magnetized or that Mr. Home previously said that his stature was about to be altered, it is not necessary to appeal to any other force than that of legerdemain or sleight of hand. Thus Mr. Robert Dale Owen states that on one occasion Miss Katie King, *alias* Mrs. White, appeared to be only eighteen inches high, but in a few seconds raised herself to her full height. We all know the history of Mr. Owen's delusions in regard to this medium, and though we have not yet actually convicted Mr. Home as thoroughly as we have Mrs. White, the time is probably not far distant when the mechanism of his elongations and contractions will be as fully exposed as were hers. A not very complex mechanism would enable a performer to increase or diminish his stature at will, and a tall man by an imperceptible flexure of the joints and curving of the back, and an equally inappreciable extension, can very readily vary his height four inches or more.

But the saints did far more astounding things with their bodies than Mr. Home with all his spiritual aid has ever ventured to attempt. Görres'* states that the blessed Ida, of Louvain, who lived in the convent of Rosenthal, was so filled with the desire to render herself acceptable to the Lord, that one night as she occupied a bed with a very devout nun, her intense longing so filled her soul that very soon all the members of her body began to swell and quickly assumed monstrous proportions. The skin of one of her legs burst, so great was the strain, and she ever afterwards had the cicatrix. The poor nun, her bed-fellow, did not know what to think of this enormous amplification of the saintly Ida, and her situation was rendered in addition, physically uncomfortable, for the swelling Ida went on enlarging, till she occupied all but a very narrow strip of the bed. Suddenly, however, things changed. Ida's body diminished little by little, till at last it was reduced to an extremely minute size. This phenomenon was reproduced, as she was returning from the church with her friend.

Here we have the evidence of a devout woman in support of the alleged miraculous event, and the testimony is as good as any adduced in favor of Mr. Home's elongations.

Levitation or rising in the air. As an instance of this performance by Mr. Home, I quote the following account by Lord Lindsay.† After mentioning Mr. Home's ability to

* La Mystique divine, naturelle et diabolique. Paris, 1861, t 1, p. 349.

† *The Spiritual Magazine.* August 1, 1871. p. 380.

discover a magnet in the dark, the noble spiritualist continues.

"I may mention that on another occasion I was sitting with Mr. Home, Lord Adare, and a cousin of his. During the sitting Mr. Home went into a trance and in that state was carried out of the window in the room next to where we were and was brought in at our window. The distance between the windows was about seven feet six inches, and there was not the slightest foot-hold between them nor was there more than a twelve inch projection to each window, which served as a ledge to put flowers on.

"We heard the window in the next room lifted up and almost immediately after we saw Home floating in the air outside our window.

"The moon was shining full into the room; my back was to the light, and I saw the shadow on the wall of the window-sill and Home's feet about six inches above it. He remained in this position for a few seconds and then glided into the room, feet foremost, and sat down.

"Lord Adare then went into the next room to look at the window from which he had been carried. It was raised about eighteen inches, and he expressed his wonder how Mr. Home had been taken through so narrow an aperture.

"Home said (still in a trance), 'I will show you,' and then, with his back to the window, he leaned back and was shot out of the aperture head first with the body rigid and then returned quite quietly.

"The window is about seventy feet from the ground. I very much doubt whether any skilful tight-rope dancer would like to attempt a feat of this description, when the only means of crossing would be by a perilous leap, or being borne across in such a manner as I have described, placing aside the question of the light."

The foregoing account is sufficient to indicate the nature of the claim put forward in behalf of Mr. Home's ability to raise himself in the air without extraneous aid. Now, let us see from the intrinsic evidence afforded by Lord Lindsay's report whether or not it is proven that Mr. Home really did pass from one window to the other as described, and if so, whether the movement was really effected by the agency of spirits.

Before the present spiritual era it was asserted by many persons, or claimed for them by credulous adherents, that they had been lifted from the ground without the aid of material agencies. It is contended by the spiritualists that these cases are similar in character and due to the same cause as those now declared to be quite common. An inquiry into the history of these earlier instances will serve to enlighten us relative to those of our own time.

According to Philostratus,* Apollonius saw the Brahmins of India rise in the air to the height of two cubits and walk there without earthly support.

The authority is not very reliable, but the Brahmins are well known to be prëeminent in feats of legerdemain. A few years ago I saw a Colonel Stodare, who had resided in India and was exhibiting his skill in magic at Egyptian Hall, London, cause a female confederate to remain in the air after a table on which she was reclining had been removed. Long wands were passed through the air above and below her without any sup

* Vita Apollonii Tyaneus, lib. iii., cap. xx. 17.

port being detected other than a slender cane which she held in one hand and which rested lightly on the floor. The trick is quite a common one among the Brahmins, and was probably used to impress Apollonius, who was regarded as a god by his followers. The instance, however, is quoted by several spiritualistic writers as establishing the possibility of levitation.

In a work on Spiritualism * by an anonymous writer, published a few years ago, I find the following statement, which, however, is taken from "Howitt's History of the Supernatural." (Vol. I., p. 491, Am. ed.)

"Savonarola, before his tragical death at the stake, and while absorbed in devotion, was seen to remain suspended at a considerable height from the floor of his dungeon. 'The historical evidence of this fact,' says Elihu Rich in the 'Encyclopedia Metropolitana,' 'is admitted by his recent biographer.'"

I suppose the "recent biographer" of Savonarola here referred to is Mr. R. R. Madden, who makes the observation stated, but whose authority for so doing can scarcely be regarded as very great. But the most recent as well as most thorough and reliable history of this great man, is that of Villari, † and this is what he says of Savonarola's last night in prison. If any such incident as levitation had occurred, Villari would certainly have referred to it.

"The night was already far advanced when he returned to

* Planchette, or the Despair of Science, being a full account of Modern Spiritualism, etc. Boston, 1869, p. 207.

† La Storia di Girolamo Savonarola, e di suoi Tempi. Firenze, 1859-1861. A translation of this work in two volumes, by Leonard Horner, was published in London in 1863.

his prison; sleep and weariness so overpowered him that almost as a sign of love and gratitude, he laid his head on the knees of the good Nicolini and soon fell into a short and light slumber, during which he appeared to smile and dream, so great was the serenity of his mind and soul." (Vol. II., p. 204).

The rest of the night was passed in prayer.

Now there is not a word here about being carried up from the floor. Some person may have made the assertion quoted by Madden and the author of *Planchette;* but Villari, who is Professor of History in the University of Pisa, evidently discredits any such story. Savonarola may at times have entertained such a delusion, for he was of a highly nervous temperament and claimed that he was subject to visions which he imagined were real events. He had read and re-read those parts of the Bible which treat of visions, angels, and apparitions, his mind had been strongly impressed with their truth, and his nervous temperament was agitated to an extreme degree. The dreams and visions of his childhood were multiplied, they constantly obtruded themselves upon his mind, and at night he was scarcely ever free from them. Thus, as Villari remarks, "he passed whole nights on his knees in his cell, a prey to visions, by which he more and more exhausted his strength, continually excited his brain, and then ended by seeing in everything a revelation from the Lord." *

If, therefore, Savonarola had entertained the delusion that he was at times lifted from the floor, there would have been nothing surpr sing in the circumstance; yet there is no credi

* *Op. cit.*, Vol. i. p. 295.

ble evidence, Mr. Elihu Rich, Mr. Howitt, the author of *Planchette*, and the "recent biographer" to the contrary, notwithstanding, that he ever had this delusion.*

No one has done more to perpetuate the stories of saints rising in the air than Calmet,† and his statements are accepted at the present day by the too willing followers of spiritualism without the least hesitation or inquiry, and generally at second or even third hand. Calmet was born in the year 1672, and lived, therefore, at a period when a belief in the supernatural was general. His education in the church did not by any means tend to lessen the force of the credulity implanted in him by nature. Thus his work shows that he believed in magic and sorcery, witchcraft, familiars, spirits, elves, demons, vampires, the possibility of a man being in two places at the same time, that the bodies of excommunicated persons do not decay, etc. He credited in full the accusations made against Gaufridi—to which we will hereafter more fully allude—and approved of his punishment. The instances he adduces in support of all his beliefs are numerous and perfectly convincing to those who are willing to accept any statement which appeals to their love for the marvellous, without asking for the proof.

* The statement comes originally from Mr. Rich, who makes it without giving the name of his authority. It is contained in a section signed with his initials in "*The Occult Sciences; Sketches of the Traditions and Superstitions of Past Times and the Marvels of the Present.* London, 1855, p. 202. A work written by himself, Rev. Edward Lindley, W. Cooke Taylor, LL.D., and Mr. Henry Thompson. I have consulted several biographers of Savonarola without finding any reference to the circumstance he relates.

† The Phantom World, or the Philosophy of Spirits, Apparitions, etc., by Augustin Calmet. Edited, with an introduction and notes, by Rev. Henry Christmas. London, 1830.

What he says in regard to the human body rising in the air comes under the same category, and has no evidence in its power stronger than that brought forward in support of his other views of supernatural phenomena.

The twenty-first chapter of his treatise is thus entitled: "Reasons which prove the possibility of Sorcerers and Witches being translated to the Sabbath." After referring to instances in the Bible, he says:

"We have in history several instances of persons full of religion and piety, who, in the fervor of their visions, have been taken up into the air, and remained there some time. We have known a good monk, who rises sometimes from the ground, and remains suspended without wishing it, without seeking to do so, especially on seeing some devotional image or hearing some devout prayer, such as *Gloria in excelsis Deo!* I know a nun to whom it has often happened to see herself thus raised up in the air to a certain distance from the earth. It was neither from choice nor from any wish to distinguish herself, since she was truly confused at it." It is not stated by Calmet that either of these instances was witnessed by him. He then innocently inquires:

"Was it by the ministrations of angels, or by the artifice of the seducing spirit who wished to inspire her with sentiments of vanity? or was it the natural effect of divine love, or fervor of devotion in these persons?"

"I do not observe that the ancient fathers of the desert, who were so spiritual, so fervent, and so great in prayer, experienced similar ecstasies."

As Calmet remarks, the phenomena were only met with in the "new saints."

Of these "new saints," who have been lifted up by unseen powers, he gives the following list:

St. Philip Neri.

St. Catharine Columbina.

St. Ignatius Loyola.

St. Robert de Paientin.

St. Bernard Ptolomæi.

St. Philip Benitas.

St. Cajetanus.

St. Alber of Sicily.

St. Dominic.

St. Christina, who was raised up after death, was restored to life, and who was thereafter so light that she could run with great swiftness.

A nun, named Seraphina, in whom the tendency to rise was so great that six sisters could not hold her down.

St. Dunstan, Archbishop of Canterbury, who, it will be recollected, caught the devil by the nose with a pair of red-hot pincers, and at whose instigation, or at least connivance, Elgiva, the wife of Edwy, was so cruelly murdered.

St. Richard, abbot of St. Vanne de Verdun.

Father Dominic Carme Dechaux, who floated in the air, and who, while in this position, was so light that he was blown about like a soap bubble.

It would be a needless piece of labor to search through the lives of the saints for the details of these asserted examples of levitation. They all rest upon the same kind of evidence, where there is any at all—the declaration of the subjects themselves, or of some of their followers. I have, therefore selected a few of the most notable instances for more thorough investigation than Calmet thought it necessary to give.

St. Philip Neri, born in 1595. Of this saint, Butler * says: "Gallonio testifies that the divine love so much dilated the breast of our saint in an extraordinary rapture, that the gristle which joined the fourth and fifth ribs on the left side was broken, which accident allowed the heart and large vessels more play."

After this statement we are prepared for any thing—and need not, therefore, be surprised that "Gallonio mentions several extraordinary raptures with which the saint was favored in prayer, and testifies that his body was sometimes seen raised from the ground during his devotions some yards high, at which times his countenance appeared shining with a bright light."

To this account Butler † appends the following remarks in the form of a note:

"We find the same authentically attested of many other servants of God. St. Ignatius Loyola was sometimes seen raised in prayer two feet above the ground, his body at the same time shining like light. The like elevations are related in the lives of St. Dominic, St. Dunstan, St. Philip Benitas, St. Cajetan, St. Albert of Sicily, B. Bernard Ptolomœi, institutor of the congregation of our Lady of Mount Olivet, Aug. xxi., B. Robert of Palentin, Aug. xviii. in the Bollandists, of St. Francis of Assisium in his life by Chalippi, and others. Many of the authors of these lives, persons of undoubted veracity,

* Lives of the Primitive Fathers, Martyrs, and other Principal Saints Compiled from Original Monuments and other Authentic Records. By the Rev. Alban Butler. Third edition. Edinburgh, 1799, vol. v., p. 345.

† *Op. cit.*, p. 348.

testify that they were eye-witnesses of these facts. Others were so careful and diligent writers that their authority cannot be questioned."

Butler cites several of the cases on the authority of Calmet, whom he praises in the highest terms. But, as showing the difficulty with which he has accepted the truth, yet not perceiving that he is using a two-edged sword, he says:

"Ennapius, a Platonic philosopher, who, in 380, wrote the lives of Porphyrius and Jamblichus, relates that the latter was often raised ten cubits into the air, and was seen surrounded with a bright light." But he denounces Ennapius as "credulous, malicious, and unworthy of credit," as being inimical to Christianity, and in fact as bad as Porphyrius and Jamblichus themselves. I am, nevertheless, decidedly of the opinion that the evidence in favor of the levitation of Jamblichus, the Neoplatonic philosopher, is fully as strong as that adduced on the side of any Christian saint, monk, nun, or medium.

Among the instances mentioned by Calmet is that of St. Theresa. This remarkable woman was born in 1515. From a very early age she was afflicted with frequent fits of fainting and violent pain at her heart, which sometimes deprived her of her senses; sharp pains were frequent through her whole frame, her sinews began to shrink up, and finally, in August 1537, when she was in her twenty-third year, she fell into a lethargic coma or trance, which lasted four days. At one time she was thought to be dead, and her grave was actually dug. During this attack she bit her tongue in several places, and was for a long time unable to swallow; sometimes her whole body seemed as if her bones were disjointed in every part and her head was in extreme disorder and pain.

As Madden * remarks, from whom these particulars are taken, though they are found in Butler,† and in her autobiography: "It is impossible for a medical man to read this account of the occasional falling into a lethargic state, fits of fainting and swooning, violent spasms, pain at the heart, temporary loss of reason, shrinking of the sinews, oppression, with a profound sense of sadness, biting of the tongue in many places when out of her senses, inability to swallow any liquid, distortion of the whole frame as if all her bones were disjointed, subsequent inability to stir hand or foot for some time, and a generally-diffused soreness so as to be unable to bear being touched, without coming to the conclusion that the sufferer labored under physical disease of a low nervous or gastric kind, with continu ous fever probably complicated with epileptic tendencies."

There can be no doubt that she was of a highly hysterical temperament, and was subject to paroxysms of hysterical chorea, catalepsy, and epilepsy. Her visions became very frequent, and her raptures were even more numerous. In rapture, as she says, "the body loses all the use of its voluntary functions and every part remains in the same posture, without feeling, hearing or seeing, at least so as to perceive it."

During these raptures she was at times under the impression that she was raised in the air. Speaking of the elevation of her soul, she says:

"Sometimes my whole body was carried with it so as to be raised up from the ground, though this was seldom. When I

* Phantasmata; or Illusions and Fanaticisms of Protean Forms, productive of Great Evils. London, 1857. vol. i., p. 1818.

† *Op. cit.*, vol. x., p. 324, *et seq.*

had a mind to resist these raptures, there seemed to me somewhat of a mighty force under my feet, which raised me up, that I knew not what to compare it to." *

It is said, Bishop Ypres saw her thus lifted up. The instance in question is similar in general features to all the others recorded of enthusiastic saints and other religious persons. The organization of St. Theresa was such as to allow of her imagining anything as reality; and the hallucination of being lifted up, as I shall show hereafter, is one of the most common, experienced by ecstatics.

A case not referred to by Calmet is that of St. Francis of Assisium, whose life is contained in Butler's† collection. This self-denying and enthusiastic saint died in 1226. He constantly wore a hair-shirt, rarely ate anything cooked, and, when he did, put ashes and water on it, slept on the ground with a piece of wood or stone for a pillow, never drank enough water to satisfy his thirst, when tormented by an occasional accession of sexual desire, stripped himself and rolled in the snow, and made large snow-balls which he clasped in his arms, imagined that during a state of exaltation he had been marked in the hands, feet and side in imitation of the wounds received by Christ during the crucifixion, and exhibited the scars—the stigmata of catalepsy—besides giving many other evidences of laboring under mental derangement. Among his miracles, was that of curing a man of a virulent ulcer of the face by kissing the sore. It is therefore not strange that levitation was among his powers. As Butler says: "The raptures and other extraordinary favors which he received from God in contempla-

* Butler, *Op. cit.*, vol. x., p. 359. † Id. p. 71.

tion, he was careful to conceal from men. St. Bonaventure and other writers of his life assure us that he was frequently raised from the ground in prayer. F. Leo, his secretary and confessor, testified that he had seen him in prayer raised from the ground so high, that his disciple could only touch his feet, which he held and watered with his tears, and that sometimes he was raised much higher."* As F. Leo is shown by this extract to have been of an excitable and nervous temperament, we would scarcely be warranted in placing implicit confidence in any statement he might make bordering on affirmation of a miraculous act.

But the most credulous writer relating to supernatural qualities and performances of the saints is Görres† some of whose examples have just been cited and to whom I shall frequently have to refer. The case of St. Thomas of Villanova, detailed by him, exhibits in a striking light the nervous organization of the levitants, and I therefore quote it in the present connection.

St. Thomas, of Villanova, was the subject, it appears, of continual attacks of ecstacy when preaching, praying or saying mass. One day he was preaching at Valladolid before the Emperor Charles V. on the washing of feet (not a bad subject for the Saints of those days), when he repeated the words of St. Peter : "Lord, dost thou wash my feet?" In explaining these he said : "Thou Lord to me? Thou my God, the glory of the angels, the ornament of heaven, the master of all creation!

* *Op. cit.*, p. 104.

†La Mystique divine, naturelle, et diabolique. Ouvrage traduit de l'Allemand par M. Charles Sainte Foi. Deuxieme édition, Paris, 1861.

Thou to me?" As he pronounced these last words "to me" he stopped suddenly and became as immovable as a marble statue. His eyes were raised towards heaven, his tears flowed, and he was unable to say another word. This often happened to him, and when he was seized while in the pulpit, the congregation waited a half hour, and more even, till he had come to himself. Priests and laity were equally anxious to hear him preach, for they knew that in these conditions he spoke as an angel from heaven, and singularly touched those who heard him. But for fear of being considered a saint he ceased preaching. Nevertheless the more he fled from glory the more it pursued him. One Easter morning as he was walking in the corridors of the Archiepiscopal palace with his chaplain Bovello repeating his Breviary, at the words *Et videntibus illis, elevatus est,*" he was seized with ecstasy and carried up from the ground, remaining suspended in the air from six o'clock in the morning until five in the evening. A great number of persons in and out of the house came to see him in that state.

St. Thomas explained the event by saying that, just as he began to chant the anthem "*videntibus illis,*" a troop of angels took up the words and him also, and that the music was so ravishingly beautiful that he was deprived for the time of the use of his senses.

Görres cites several other examples not referred to by Calmet.

Thus Maria d'Agréda was often elevated above the ground in the communion or even when reading passages relating to the grandeur and goodness of God. The music of the Church was equally sufficient to put her into this condition, which generally lasted about three hours. Margaret of Hungary was also raised from the earth after the annunciation. St. Agnes was one day found by a sister in her cell on her knees and raised several inches from the floor.

Caeson of Heisterbach knew a priest who every time he said mass was lifted up a foot in the air, from the beginning of the service to the communion.

Görres gives a list of twenty-two others by name, which he states is not complete, who have been lifted up sometimes in view of large numbers of people, remaining thus suspended for several hours.

St. Peter, of Alcantara, while saying his breviary on the high road, was elevated in the air in this position several feet above the earth, was seen by many travellers, who waited till he had regained his senses in order that they might receive his blessing. The Saint, however, overpowered with humility, came down and ran away as fast as he could.

On another occasion he was carried up in the air to a great height, far above the trees, when with his arms crossed on his chest he continued to soar, while hundreds of little birds gathered around him, making a most agreeable concert with their songs.

St. Esperance, of Brenegalla, was still more greatly honored, for once, when she was praying in church, she was elevated in the air, where she was seen soaring with the infant Jesus in her arms!

Sometimes, as Görres declares, it is impossible to cause the levitants to descend. Thus the blessed Gilles, while one day reading a passage relative to ecstasy, was lifted up above the table. When found in this state by some of the brethren he was seized and pulled at with all their strength, but they could not get him down.

On Ascension day, Agnes, of Bohemia, as related in an old manuscript, while walking in the garden of the convent with her two sisters singing pious songs, was suddenly raised from the earth and carried without any visible help up to the clouds, so that she disappeared from sight. Her sisters ceased their song, and filled with admiration fixed their eyes towards heaven, and with tears waited for Agnes to return. At the end of an hour she re-appeared; they asked her where she had been and what had happened to her; but they could obtain no other answer than a sweet and amiable smile. "She had," says Görres, "contemplated the secrets of God which no one is permitted to reveal."

The ecstatic paroxysm was sometimes so powerful with Dominic de Jésus-Marie that he was raised up to the ceiling of his cell, where he remained without earthly support for a day and a night. There were sceptics in those days as well as in our own, and many of the ungodly in Valencia ridiculed the idea of levitation as asserted to be constantly realized in the church of that city. One of the scoffers was bold enough, while Dominic was floating around, to seize him by the feet; but he was borne on high, and being frightened let go and fell to the earth. After suffering great pain for his temerity, he was constrained to admit the truth of the elevation.

The cases cited are attributed to the influence of the Holy Spirit or of angels. There is another class of examples supposed to be due to the agency of demons, witches, or other diabolical power. Thus those who had made a compact with the devil always went to the Sabbath by supernatural agencies, and generally through the air astride of a broomstick.* Others are cited by Mather.† And many are contained in treatises on the "black art." The evidence in support of this category of instances is fully as strong as that in favor of the more orthodox variety.

A very well authenticated case—as authentication goes in such matters—is that "*concerning the witchcraft practised by Jane Brooks, upon Richard Jones, son of Henry Jones, of Shepton Mallet.*‡ Among other spells laid on this unfortunate youth we are told that:

"On the 25th of February, between two and three in the afternoon, the boy being at the house of Richard Ifles, in Shepton Mallet, went out of the room into the garden. Ifles his wife followed him, and was within two yards when she saw him rise up from the ground before her, and so mounted higher and higher till he passed in the air over the garden wall and was carried on above ground more than thirty years [yards ?], falling at last at one Jordan's door at Shepton, where he was found as dead for a time, but coming to himself told

* Many of the older works on sorcery and witchcraft contain plates representing the departure to the Sabbath and the orgies which there took place under the auspices of the devil. Among the most striking are the "*Description de l'assemblée des sorciers qu'on appelle Sabbat*" in "*L'Histoire des imaginations extravagants de Monsieur Oufle,*" Paris 1754, t. ii. and "*Départ pour le Sabbat,*" and other plates in the second edition of the Dictionnaire Infernale, Paris, 1826.

† Magnolia Christi Americana, etc. First American from the London edition of 1702. Hartford, 1720.

‡ Sadducismus Triumphatus, or a Full and Plain Evidence concerning Witches and Apparitions. By Joseph Glanvil: London, 1726, p. 285 et seq.

Jordan that Jane Brocks had taken him up by the arm out of Ifles' garden and carried him in the air as narrated." It is perhaps scarcely necessary to add that Jane Brooks was condemned and executed.

This same Joseph Glanvil, who was chaplain in ordinary to King Charles II., and like some equally credulous persons of the present day, a Fellow of the Royal Society, reports * another case on the very bad authority of Mr. Valentine Greatrix, or Greatrakes, the notorious healer by laying on of hands. In this instance, a butler, who asserted that he was visited by a spectre, was shut up in a room with several persons, in order that he might not be carried off as the spectre had threatened. While together in the room, he was perceived to rise from the ground, and, notwithstanding that Mr. Greatrix "and another lusty man," caught hold of him and held him with all their strength, he was forcibly taken up, and for a considerable time floated about in the air over their heads. At length he fell and was caught in the arms of his guardians.

It would be very easy to go on and quote numerous other instances of levitation both of ancient and modern times, of sacred and diabolical agency, but the foregoing are sufficient to show the character of the evidence on which they rest. By such testimony anything could be proved, no matter what the degree of absurdity or of opposition to physical laws.

In all supposed instances of levitation such as have been cited, the true explanation may be given by referring them to one or other of the following causes.

1. *An hallucination on the part of the subject, characterized by*

* *Op. cit.*, p. 356.

the sensation of rising in the air, or of flying, and illusion on the part of those asserting themselves to have been witnesses.

A. De Boismont * remarks : "The sensation of flying is rather common ; frequently in dreams we feel ourselves carried along with the rapidity of an arrow; we accomplish great distances just lightly touching the ground. We have noticed this fact in a literary man of our acquaintance, whom we have several times found with fixed eyes, and who said to us, 'I am flying, do not stop me.' On returning to himself he described his sensations, and it seemed to him that he really had flown. This sensation was experienced as far back as the time of St. Jerome, who relates that frequently in his dreams he felt himself flying over mountains, seas, etc."

Turning again to Görres, that mine of wealth of alleged supernatural phenomena, we find that with Beatrix of Nazareth, during her ecstatic paroxysms, it seemed to her in the night, that she flew in the air. St. Joseph of Copertin, being in ecstasy, appeared to brother Junipero to be as light as straw.

Oringa, on coming out of a paroxysm, felt her body to be so light and agile, that she was obliged to touch it with her fingers to make sure that it was still present.

Madame d'Arnim, Goethe's friend, in speaking of the sensation in question, says: 'I was certain that I flew and floated in the air. By a simple, elastic pressure of the toe, I was in the air. I floated silently and deliciously at two or three feet above the earth: I alighted, mounted again, I flew from side to side, and then returned. A few days after, I was taken with

* A History of Dreams, Visions, Apparitions, Ecstasy, Magnetism and Somnambulism. American Edition. Philadelphia: 1855, p. 94.

fever. I went to bed and slept. It happened two weeks after I was confined.' *

Numerous other instances of similar cases are recorded in works on psychological medicine, and several have come under my own observation.

In one of these, a lady, of strongly-marked hysterical temperament, and of most fanatical religious tendencies, imagined that she was frequently raised from the ground while in the act of saying her prayers. She usually spent several hours each day in these exercises, and during the whole time was in a state of fervid exaltation, which rendered her insensible to all that was passing around her. While in this condition, she would exclaim, "I rise, I rise! I see angels!" and, with her hands raised on high, her head elevated, her face turned upward, and her countenance illuminated with ecstatic radiance, she really did seem, to some superficial and sympathetic ob servers, to be lifted up. Among others, her maid was strongly convinced that the elevation was actual; but stronger-minded members of her family could see nothing of the kind, and eventually the lady herself became convinced that she was the victim of self-deception. A young married lady, formerly under my professional care, was very confident that, during the cataleptic seizures to which she was subject, she was raised from her bed, and she appealed with confidence to those surrounding her to confirm her statements. It almost always happened that some one present expressed the opinion that she really was lifted up several inches.

In another case, occurring in a young and strongly hyster-

* Correspondence de Goethe et de Bettina. Translated by M. Sebact Albin. t. i., p. 68.

ical, unmarried lady, the sensation of lightness is at times so powerfully felt, that she is sure she is floating in the air. This lady is a believer in spiritualism, and is firmly convinced that, at these periods of lightness, her soul has left its body. She recovers her weight with a long drawn sigh of relief, that she has returned to the right dwelling-place, and is conscious during her ecstasies of a fear that she may never get back.

Such a misfortune is really said, according to Pliny,* to have happened to Hermotinus, the Clazomenian, who seemed frequently to have his body deserted by his soul, and as if it had wandered about in the world. At the return of it, he would relate things which had been seen or performed at such a distance that no one could talk of them, unless, he had been present. These things he did for a long time to the great admiration of those among whom he lived. At last, however, being in one of his trances, his enemies seized upon his body and burnt it, by which proceeding the returning soul was disappointed of its usual place of residence and retreat.

It is also affirmed that Johannes Scotus, the philosopher, used to go into trances, so that he would sit sometimes for the space of a whole day immovable, his mind and senses bound up or wandering far off from his body. One day when his soul was thus roaming over the earth, or perhaps to other spheres as the saying is, his body was taken by some who were unacquainted with his peculiarity, and buried so deeply in the earth that the soul could never find it again.

The majority of cases met with in the lives of saints belong to the category of disease. Nearly all the subjects were the

* Historia Naturalis Tarvisii. 1479. Lib. VII. c. lii.

victims of some severe disorder of the nervous system, by which they were rendered peculiarly susceptible to hallucinations; and their more ardent followers were either similarly affected or were so impressed by the power of suggestion, already considered in this essay, as to be fit recipients of erroneous mental or sensorial impressions.

The appearance as if about to fly is very common in cases of ecstasy, and is due to the raising of the arms, the upward look, and the elevation of the body on the extreme points of the toes. This position is sometimes kept for hours, and may readily—as the stature is increased in height—lead to the opinion that the body is off the ground, especially in the cases of women whose feet cannot readily be seen, owing to the drapery of their dress.

A sensation as if the body were passing rapidly through the air is induced by certain drugs, particularly aconite.

2. *Unintentional exaggeration, misinterpretation, and inaccuracy of statement.* It frequently happens that, during hysterical convulsions, the affected person makes strong efforts to rise, which attempts are strenuously resisted by the by-standers. In former times when every seizure of the kind was regarded as being directly due to the agency of demons or other supernatural beings acting either within the sufferer (possession) or from without (obsession) the idea was very naturally entertained that but for the assistance of friends at hand, severe injury would result from the convulsive movements. When therefore, the limbs were thrown about, or the body writhed, or he tongue was bitten, the afflicted epileptic, cataleptic, or hysterical individual was at once seized, and the statement made than all the phenomena of the paroxysm were caused by some kind of

spiritual power. At the same time the actual violence of the manifestations was always over-estimated, just as is invariably done by spectators of our own day. It thus often happened that a contortion of the body was regarded as an effort of a demon to rend it or carry it off. No sensible person can read the accounts of witchcraft which have come down to us, and to which fuller reference will presently be made, without being convinced that this was a frequent interpretation of well-known pathological symptoms, or doubt that several of the asserted instances of levitation—as for instance that of sister Seraphina—are to be explained in a similar manner.

3. *Insufficient evidence.* Most of the instances of levitation which have been recorded rest on insufficient evidence—such as would be inadequate to establish the fact in a court of law. This is the case, for example, in several of those said to have occurred in the persons of saints, monks and nuns. It does not appear that Calmet ever saw the human body lifted up without material agency, although he refers to several cases of which he had heard. Hearsay testimony is of so equivocal a character as to be disregarded in all matters of importance, and yet we are expected to rely on it as sufficient to establish the fact of miraculous events, which, of all others, should require the most unerring and irrefragable demonstration.

Take, for example, the alleged elevation of Savonarola, which is quoted with peculiar unction by the spiritualists of the present day. Research shows that the story is altogether of comparatively recent origin, and that its truth has been assumed by interested believers in supernaturalism, without due pains being taken to verify its accuracy.

And so, relative to St. Ignatius Loyola, whose elevation in

the air is also a *point d'appui* for the spiritualists. A recent biographer, a sincere and devout member of the Roman Catholic Church, thus speaks of St. Ignatius and his faithful adherents, in connection with a report—the last of the kind—that a supernatural light had been seen around his body:

"His children never claimed for him a power of working prodigies, and he would certainly greatly have regretted such an attitude. All the remarkable circumstances of the kind that it has been thought right to detail may be set aside, if the reader so pleases. The true and only miracle that it is necessary to know and to appreciate is that of a most noble, extraordinary, and original character and an admirable life." *

We know that even undoubted events, when seen through the prejudiced historian's spectacles, become so changed in character as to be scarcely recognizable, and that no two persons witnessing a transaction will give precisely the same version of it. Even in so exact a science as chemistry, authorities differ, and, in testing for poisons, one observer has perceived the looked-for reaction, while another, working under the same conditions, has failed to see the change of color or the precipitation. The sensorial impressions of some persons are always modified by their mental bias.

4. *Intentional misstatement.* Some of the instances are probably due to misrepresentation, with the view of enhancing the reputation for sanctity of the subjects, or simply from that love for telling marvellous stories which is so inherent a quality with the majority of mankind; such, in all likelihood, are the earlier examples—as that of St. Dunstan.

* Ignatius Loyola and the Early Jesuits. By Stewart Rose. London,

The cases, too, recorded in connection with witchcraft are many of them clearly fraudulent in character, fabricated for the purpose of injuring some obnoxious person by the imputation of being a witch. The boy who asserted, in conjunction with the wife of Ifles, that he had been carried over a wall by one Jane Brooks, was evidently in a conspiracy with Mrs. Ifles to accomplish the destruction of an innocent woman.

5. *Legerdemain.* This explanation has already been commented upon in connection with the Brahminical exploits made before Apollonius Tyaneus; that it is sufficient to account for many cases cannot be questioned.

The modern instances, attributed directly to the influence of the spiritualists, are scarcely deserving of mention. None of them are well authenticated, and all are more reasonably explained by ascribing them to one or several of the causes specified. Performed in the dark, they afford abundant opportunity for deceit on the one part, and hallucination or illusion on the other. They do not even claim to be as powerful manifestations as those specially referred to in this essay, for the latter were asserted to be done in broad daylight, and the subjects could be touched by those present; while those of our day avoid inquiry, and are performed under such circumstances as to defy thorough examination. In one case which came under my notice, the medium, a woman, was bound in a chair and seated at one end of a long table. The lights were then extinguished, and a blanket hung over the window, so as to exclude the feeblest ray of light from a dark night. The company, *with the exception of the medium's husband,* sat around the table, holding each other's hands. The only inquirers present were myself and another gentleman, who were carefully sandwiched between the faithful, who kept up a dismal howling while the experiment went on. The husband stood at one end of the room, outside of the circle. There was a good deal of noise at the medium's end of the table, which was only partially drowned by the lugubrious singing. Suddenly she exclaimed, "Now!" The gas was turned on, and she was found seated in the middle of the table still fastened to the chair; all, present except my friend and myself, were convinced that the spirits had placed her there. We were not, for the reasons mainly, that it was entirely practicable for her husband to have put her on the table without his movements being known to us, and that it was very easy, as I have ascertained by experiment, for her to have climbed to the top of the table without any assistance whatever. Now applying the foregoing principles to the case of Mr. Home, as related by Lord Lindsay, and we perceive the possibility of:

1. *Hallucination on the part of the Narrator.* Lord Lindsay may have dined heartily; his cravat may have been too tight, or, from some other cause, the circulation of blood in his brain may been accelerated so as to have produced active congestion, or retarded so as to have caused passive congestion

It is infinitely more probable that Lord Lindsay had a hallucination than that Mr. Home was, without material aid, and in opposition to the laws of gravity, suspended in the air, and moved about in the manner stated.

2. *Unintentional exaggeration, misinterpretation and inaccuracy of statement*—Lord Lindsay says: "We heard the window in the next room lifted up, and almost immediately after, we saw Home floating in the air, outside our window."

Taking this sentence by itself, we should be led to believe

that Lord Lindsay in it, asserted the fact that *he* saw Mr. Home floating in the air; but when we come to peruse the next paragraph, we are induced to think that he saw nothing of the kind, in fact, that he was so situated that he could not see it.

"The moon was shining full into the room; *my back was to the light*, and I saw the shadow on the wall of the window sill, and Home's feet about six inches above it. He remained in this position for a few seconds, then raised the window and glided into the room, feet foremost, and sat down."

Lord Adare went into the next room to see how Mr. Home got out of the window, and he alone, so Lord Lindsay tells us, saw the second experiment.

To be sure, Lord Lindsay does say he saw Mr. Home's feet; but as the room was dark, and he had only the uncertain light of the moon to assist him in his observations, it is quite probable he was mistaken, as we are all apt to be, under similar circumstances.

3. *Insufficient evidence.*—The testimony of one person to the occurrence of so remarkable an event as the body of a man floating in the air, in opposition to the laws of gravity, cannot be regarded as sufficient to decide the matter affirmatively. The experience of the world is against the possibility of such a circumstance, and Lord Lindsay's evidence in view of the possibility of hallucination, illusion, or misinterpretation, on his part, must go for very little, if for anything at all. We know that hallucinations or illusions do occur to us all under certain circumstances; we know that we often interpret phenomena wrongly, and the probability of one or another of these conditions being the governing factor in the present instance is infinitely greater than the alternative which Lord

Lindsay would have us accept. There were three gentlemen present in the room besides Mr. Home. Lord Adare, we may admit, accepts the account given by Lord Lindsay. Indeed, he may be said to be the father of it. But why have we no word from the "cousin of his" who formed one of the company? There cannot be too much evidence on so important a point as this.

4. Lord Lindsay's character, as a gentleman, puts him above the imputation of intentional misstatement.

5. *Legerdemain.* That Lord Lindsay may have been deceived by a trick, is a supposition which has a good deal of plausibility in its support. It appears that Mr. Home in the first experiment, went into another room alone, and was from this second room brought into the other, through the window. It would have been very easy for him, while alone, to have arranged means for passing from one window to the other—if he did pass at all—and for such means to have escaped detection. Many of the examples of conjuring performances which I have cited, are far more remarkable than would have been Mr. Home's, even if he had really passed from one window to the other without *visible* material agency, as Lord Lindsay supposes.

But as these lines are being written, the true explanation comes to hand, showing that both Lord Lindsay and Lord Adare suffered from a hallucination. In an interesting paper, Dr. Carpenter,* evidently referring to this account of Lord Lindsay's, says: "A whole party of believers will affirm that

* On Fallacies of Testimony respecting the Supernatural. *Contemporary Review*, Jan., 1876.

they saw Mr. Home float out of one window and in at another, while a single honest sceptic declares that Mr. Home was sitting in his chair all the time." This "honest sceptic" is probably the cousin incidentally mentioned by Lord Lindsay. It is scarcely necessary to pursue the inquiry further.

There are perhaps fifty cases of levitation on record. I will engage to supply more and better authenticated instances of any other hitherto mentioned supernatural phenomenon; such as lizards living in the human stomach, persons walking without their heads, people with glass legs or arms, others who are coffee-pots; or to go to the very opposite, instances of the force of gravity or the power of spirits being so great as to prevent the body being raised at all.

Thus, turning again to Görres,* we find that St. Joseph of Copertino went into the state of ecstasy at any circumstance which reminded him of God. The ringing of a bell, the chanting in a church, the name of Jesus, of Mary, or of any saint, a picture of the passion of Christ, an allusion to the glory of paradise, the sight of a holy image, were sufficient any one of them to induce the condition in question; and as such occasions were in his monastic life of never-ceasing occurrence, the susceptible saint was continually passing from one trance into another. On one occasion, as he was carrying the chalice, the spell seized him and he fell at full length on the ground, holding the vessel to his breast. After some trouble, this was taken from him, but he remained stretched out on the earth as if dead, so powerfully attached to the ground that a brother named Ludovic could not raise him, and it was necessary for several

* *Op. Cit.*, t. ii. p. 19.

persons to unite all their strength in the attempt before he could be lifted up. It will be remembered that this was the same saint, who, on another occasion, was as light as a straw.

Excessive gravitation, like levitation, appears to be possessed by saints and sinners alike. Thus it is recorded by Neubrigensis, and also by Huntington,* that Raynerus, a wicked minister of a more wicked abbot, while crossing the sea with his wife, so overweighted the ship with his iniquity that in the midst of the stream it was unable to stir, at which the mariners, astonished, cast lots, and the lot fell upon Raynerus. And lest this should be thought to happen by chance they cast the lots again and again, and still the lot fell upon the same Raynerus. Whereupon they put him out of the ship, and presently the ship was as if eased of her burden, and sailed away. "Certainly," adds the pious chronicler, "a great judgment of God, and a great miracle, but yet recorded by one that is no fabulous author, saith Sir Richard Baker."

Instances of assumed excessive weight are not uncommon in the annals of hysteria, and several such, in which the patients declared they could not rise from their beds or chairs, on account of the attraction which restrained them, have come under my notice. It has repeatedly happened that these persons have succeeded in persuading their attendants and friends that they spoke the truth, and experiment has appeared to give additional sanction to their assertions.

In such cases the expectant attention of the observer causes

* The Wonders of the Little World, by Nathaniel Wanley, M. A., Vicar of Trinity Parish, London, 1806, p. 400. From Baker's Chron. p. 72.

the deception. Thus, when no metal heavier than water was known, it was not surprising that Dr. Pearson, as he poised upon his finger the first globule of potassium produced by Sir Humphrey Davy's battery, should have exclaimed "Bless me, how heavy it is!" though when thrown upon water the metal floated upon it.*

But the following story will undoubtedly be received by all earnest spiritualists as a genuine instance of excessive gravitation or adhesion caused by extra mundane interference :

"In the northern borders of England and on the other side of the river Humber, in the parish of Hovëden lived the rector of that Church with his concubine. This concubine one day sat rather imprudently on the tomb of St. Osanna, sister to king Ofred, which was made of wood and raised above the ground in the shape of a seat. When she attempted to rise from the place, her posteriors stuck to the wood in such a manner that she never could be parted from it till, in the presence of the people who ran to see her, she had suffered her clothes to be torn from her, and had received a severe discipline on her naked body and that to a great effusion of blood, and with many tears and devout supplications on her part. Which done, and after she had engaged to submit to further penance, she was divinely released." †

* Dr. Carpenter. Fallacies of Testimony respecting the Supernatural. *Contemporary Review*, Jan., 1876.

† The History of the Flagellants, otherwise of Religious Flagellations among different nations, and especially among Christians—being a Paraphrase and Commentary on the Historia Flagellantrium of the Abbé Boileau, Doctor of the Sorbonne, etc. By one who is not a Doctor of the Sorbonne [De Lolme]. The second edition, London, 1783, p. 317. The miracle referred to is quoted from the "Itinerarium Cambriæ" of Sylvester Giraldus, a native of Wales, who wrote about the year 1188.

A remedy so potent in gravitation would probably prove equally efficacicus in levitation.

Another power claimed for the physical mediums is *the ability to resist the effects of physical and chemical agents.* To enter into the consideration of all the alleged phenomena under this head would be profitless. I shall, therefore, take the most remarkable of them all; the asserted non-combustibility of the bodies of certain mediums when brought in contact with flames or intensely heated substances.

As with levitation, incombustibility goes back to a very early period. Starting with Meschach, Shadrach and Abednego, who walked about in Nebuchadnezzar's fiery furnace without being burnt, or the hairs of their heads being scorched, or even with the smell of fire remaining on them, we come to the saints of the new dispensation, and here we find, as usual, a mine of wealth in Görres' voluminous history.

Speaking of ecstatics, he says* that as they are, for the time being, above the ordinary laws of nature, they might be supposed to be removed from their influence. And, in fact, it is proved that fire, the most terrible of all the elements, has no action on them. Thus St. Catherine of Sienna, was one day seated in the kitchen occupied in turning the spit and in preparing dinner for her family. Left to her meditations, she fell into ecstasy and naturally the spit stopped. But her sister-in-law, being present, took charge of the culinary operations, and left Catherine in her trance. After the meal, when the family had gone to bed, the sister-in-law returned to the kitchen to see how Catherine was getting along, and found that she had

* *Op. cit.*, t. ii. p. 51.

fallen from the chair with her face in the midst of the burning coals on the hearth. The sister-in-law, with a cry of horror, seized Catherine and dragged her from the fire, thinking, of course, that she was severely burnt, but to her great astonishment, not only was there no injury, but there was no smell of fire about her, or even ashes sticking to her clothes.

This was not the only time that the like circumstance happened; for she was often, in presence of numerous witnesses, thrown into the fire by an invisible power. When the spectators, weeping and affrighted, endeavored to pull her from the flames, she escaped from their hands and laughing, said: "Be not afraid, it is Malatasca, (the name she gave the devil) who has done this."

Another time, being in church, near to a pillar to which were attached a number of lighted candles, one of the latter fell on her head while she was in a state of contemplation, and was not extinguished till it was entirely consumed. Upon examination, it was discovered that she was not in the least burnt, and that not even her veil was injured.

St. Simon d'Assissi, being one day in ecstasy, a burning coal fell on his foot, and remained there till it was consumed, without the saint sustaining any injury, or even feeling the heat.

In the middle ages, the ordeal of fire was frequently employed for the purpose of establishing the guilt or innocence of an accused person. Thus, in questions of state, the accused was obliged to walk over nine ploughshares heated to redness. If he did this without being injured, he was considered to be innocent of the alleged crime; but if he was burnt, his guilt was deemed to have been established, and he was punished accordingly.

Sometimes the accused walked blindfolded over and among the ploughshares laid on the ground, and at others was obliged to press each one with the naked feet. Again, the ordeal consisted in the accused person carrying in his hand for a certain distance, usually nine feet, a piece of red hot iron, the weight of which varied according to the gravity of the alleged offence.

This ordeal was employed in the determination of various doubtful questions. The count of Modena, in 996, was executed on the charge of loving the empress, wife of Otho III., the lady herself, in the fury of unrequited love, being the accuser. But after his death, the countess, before the emperor, disproved the charge against her husband by carrying the red hot iron and sustaining no injury therefrom. Otho, convinced by this test of his injustice, caused the empress to be burnt at the stake as a false witness.

The mother of two illegitimate sons of Robert, Duke of Normandy, established their paternity to the satisfaction of the alleged father by holding, unhurt, a red hot iron in her hand.

Pietro Aldrobandini, in order to show that Pietro di Pavia, Bishop of Florence was guilty of simony and heresy, offered to submit to the ordeal by fire. After imposing religious ceremonies, he walked slowly between two piles of blazing wood, ten feet long, five feet wide, and four and a half feet high; the passage between them being six feet wide and covered with an inch or two of glowing coals. The violence of the flames agitated his dress and hair, but he emerged without hurt, even the hair on his legs being unsinged, barelegged and barefooted though he was. Desiring to return through the pyre, he was prevented by the admiring crowd, who rushed around him in triumph, kissing his feet and garments and endangering his life in their transports, until he was rescued by his fellow monks. A formal statement of the facts was sent to Rome by the Florentines, the Papal court gave way, and the bishop was deposed; while the monk who had given so striking a proof of his steadfast faith, was marked for promotion and eventually died Cardinal of Albano.*

Besides the proof by the red hot iron and fire itself, there was another by boiling water, in which the hand was plunged into water heated to the boiling point. It was then wrapped in linen and sealed with the signet of the judge, to be examined on the third day. If then, the member was found to be uninjured, the accused was considered innocent, but if any evidence of the action of heat was discovered, guilt was inferred.

That such performances admitted of deceit and jugglery there is no doubt, neither is there any question but that such deceit and jugglery were often practised by those, or in the interest of those who were in favor with the authorities, or who voluntarily availed themselves of the ordeal for the purpose of accomplishing some cherished object. For many centuries preparations for making the skin and clothing incombustible have been known, and fire-eaters and other conjurors with burning coals, and excessively heated bodies, have flourished in various parts of the world. A different interpretation being given to the cause of their immunity according to the character of the performer, the bias of the reporter, or the spirit of the age in which the phenomena occurred.

* Superstition and Force. Essays on the Wager of Law, the Wager of Pattle, The Ordeal, Torture. By Henry C. Lea, Philadelphia, 1866, p. 209. Many other cases similar to the foregoing, are cited in this very learned work.

Thus Görres, who has given us so many excellent examples of the power possessed by the saints to resist fire, relates the following history of a like immunity with which one, who was possessed by a demon, was endowed, prefacing it with a theory, which if not entirely satisfactory is at least ingenious.

"When possession has attacked the more profound regions of life, it is rarely confined to the cœliac axis, but soon penetrates to the lungs, which more than any other organs of the body, are in close sympathy with the nutritive system. It then happens either that the respiratory organs are so restrained that they cannot perform their functions, or that they act with such undue force that the life of the individual is endangered. There is thus formed in the lungs a vital volcano and the chest becomes a crater from which perpetually issues a devouring fire. St. Apre, bishop and confessor, being one day at Chalons-sur-Saône, saw a young man who was possessed and from whose mouth, as from a furnace, rushed sulphurous flames. As soon as he saw the saint afar off, he became furious and tried to bite all who came near him. Everybody got out of his way, but the possessed ran towards the saint as if to seize him. But the holy man advanced without fear to the encounter with the cross in his hand, and ordered the possessed to stop. As the fiery vapor which escaped from his mouth touched the face of the saint and as the possessed tried to bite him, the bishop made over the mouth of the afflicted man, the sign of the cross, and the demon no longer being able to escape in that way went out from the body of the man in the form of a diarrhœa."

Certainly this was a most ignoble ending for the fiery spirit, but the story is instructive as showing how the faculty of incombustibility was an endowment of the whole thirty feet, more or less, of intestines belonging to the possessed, and thus establishes a marked superiority of diabolical power in this direction, over that belonging to the spirits who watch over the saints, and Mr. Home.

Strabo states that the priestesses of Diana at Castabala in Cappadocia had the power of walking uninjured over burning coals, and the Hirpi by marching over burning coals were exempted by the Roman Senate from military service, and were granted other privileges. According to Varro, their immunity was due to the use of a liniment on the soles of their feet.

Lucius Florus* states that a Syrian named Eunus, a leader of the Sicilian slaves who in the second century before Christ rebelled against their Roman masters, convinced his followers of his power by breathing sulphur and fire, and that at the same time words and flames issued out of his mouth. This performance, according to Florus, was effected by Eunus placing in his mouth a nut-shell filled with sulphur and fire and perforated at both ends, and as he spoke he breathed gently through the shell and flames were emitted with his words.

St. Jerome states that the Rabbi Barchochebas, who headed the Jews in their last revolt against the Emperor Hadrian, made them believe that he was the Messiah by vomiting flames from his mouth,† and at a latter period the Emperor Constantius was greatly alarmed when informed that one of his body guards had been breathing out fire and flames.

About the close of the seventeenth century an Englishman named Richardson created great astonishment by putting live

* Lucius Florus, lib. iii., Bellum servile.

† Bayle's Dictionary, i., p. 450, art. Barchochebas.

coals into his mouth, pouring melted lead on his tongue, and swallowing melted glass.*

A hundred years later a native of Toledo, Spain, excited the wonder of Paris by similar though even more striking experiments. Thus at the School of Medicine, before the professors and three hundred students, in broad daylight, after thorough examination he performed the following feats:

1st. A vessel containing oil heated to 85° Reaumur (about 223° F.) being prepared he opened his hand and applied the palm of it several times to the oil; he then washed his face in the oil and applied the soles of his feet to it. At the end of the experiments the heat of the oil was still from 76° to 78° R. or nearly that of boiling water.

2nd. A bar of iron, from eighteen to twenty inches long and two and a half inches in breadth was brought to a cherry-red heat at one of its extremities and placed on bricks. The Spaniard then put the sole of his foot on the red part; a portion of the oil which still adhered to it at once inflamed. He then applied the other sole in like manner, and this he repeated several times.

3d. The flat part of a large iron spatula, eighteen inches in length, was brought to a cherry-red heat. The Spaniard thrust out his tongue and applied it to the red part several times.

4th. He took a lighted candle and drew the flame of it several times over the posterior part of his leg from the heel to the hip.

He was examined after these trials and no part of his skin

* Beckmann, *Op. et lo. Cit.*, p. 121.

appeared to be in the least altered. His pulse, however, had increased from 75 to 145 per minute.*

A few years afterwards another mountebank, calling himself the miraculous Spaniard, opened an exhibition in Paris where he walked barefooted on red hot iron, drew red hot bars of iron across his face, arms, and tongue, dipped his hands in melted lead, and swallowed a glass of boiling oil.

But as long ago as two hundred years these *saludores*, as they were called, were regarded as impostors, for one of them having pretended that he could endure unharmed the heat of a kindled oven, was forced by the sceptical populace into one before he had time to prepare himself for the performance, and on opening it at the end of an hour the *saludor* was found to be calcined.

Beckmann† states that when in September, 1765, he visited the copper works at Arvestad, one of the workmen, for a little drink-money, took some of the melted copper in his hand, and after showing it, threw it against the wall. He then squeezed the fingers of his horny hand close to each other, put it a few minutes under his armpit to make it sweat as he said, and taking it out again drew it over a ladle filled with melted copper, some of which he skimmed off, and moved his hand backward and forward by way of ostentation. During this performance there was a smell like that of singed horn or leather, but his hand was not burnt. The workmen in the Swedish smelting works showed the same thing to some travellers in the seventeenth century, for Regnard saw it in 1681 at the copper works in Lapland.

* Journal de Physique. Messidor, An. 11 (1803).
† *Op. Cit.*, p. 122.

Passing over the fire-eaters etc. of our own time, who do not assume that their feats are anything more than tricks of legerdermain, we come to the performances with fire which are pretended to owe their success to spiritual agency.

In the March (1868) number of *Human Nature*, Mr. Jencken, quoted by Mr. Home,* thus writes: "Mr. Home (after various manifestations) then continued, 'we have gladly shown you our power over fluids, we will now show you our power over solids.' He then knelt down before the hearth, and deliberately breaking up a glowing piece of coal in the fire place, took up a largish lump of incandescent coal and placing the same in his left hand, proceeded to explain that the caloric had been extracted by a process known to them, (the spirits) and that the heat could in part be returned. This he proved by alternately cooling and heating the coal; and to convince us of the fact, allowed us to handle the coal which had become cool, then suddenly resumed its heat sufficient to burn one, as I again touched it. I examined Mr. Home's hand, and quite satisfied myself that no artificial means had been employed to protect the skin, which did not even retain the smell of smoke. Mr. Home then re-seated himself, and having described how the waters in the decanters were to be used, awoke from his trance quite pale and exhausted."

Again, Mr. Wallace † says: "But perhaps the best attested and most extraordinary phenomenon connected with Mr. Home's mediumship, is what is called the fire test. In a state of trance he takes a glowing coal from the hottest part of a

* Incidents in My Life, second series. New York, 1872, p. 182.

† On Miracles and Modern Spiritualism. Three Essays: London, 1875, p. 159.

bright fire, and carries it round the room so that every one may see and feel that it is a real one. This is testified by Mr. H. D. Jencken, Lord Lindsay, Lord Adare, Miss Douglas, Mr. S. C. Hall, and many others. But more strange still, he can detect the same power in other persons or convey it to them. A lump of red hot coal was once placed on Mr. S. C. Hall's head in the presence of Lord Lindsay, and of other persons. Mrs. Hall, in a communication to the Earl of Dunraven (given in the *Spiritual Magazine*, 1870, p. 178), says: Mr. Hall was seated nearly opposite to where I sat, and I saw Mr. Home after standing about half a minute at the back of Mr. Hall's chair, deliberately place the lump of burning coal on his head! I have often wondered that I was not frightened, but I was not; I had perfect faith that he would not be injured. Some one said, 'Is it not hot?' Mr. Hall answered, 'Warm, but not hot.' Mr. Home had moved a little way, but returned, still in a trance; he smiled and seemed quite pleased, and then proceeded to draw up Mr. Hall's white hair over the red coal. The white hair had the appearance of silver thread over the red coal. Mr. Home drew the hair into a sort of pyramid, the coal still red showing beneath the hair.

"When taken off the head without in the slightest degree injuring it, or singeing the hair, others attempted to touch the coal and were burnt. Lord Lindsay and Miss Douglas have also had hot coals placed in their hands, and describe them as feeling rather cold than hot; though at the same time they burn any one else, and even scorch the face of the holder if approached too closely. The same witnesses also testify that Mr. Home has placed red-hot coals inside his waistcoat, and has put his face into the middle of the fire, his hair falling into the flames, yet not being in the least singed. The same power of resisting fire can be temporarily given to inanimate objects. Mr. H. Nisbet of Glasgow states (*Human Nature, Feb.* 1870) that in his own house in Jan. 1870, Mr. Home placed a red-hot coal in the hands of a lady and gentleman to whom it only felt warm; and then placed the same on a folded newspaper, burning a hole through eight layers of paper. He then took a fresh and blazing coal and laid it on the same newspaper, carrying it about the room for three minutes, when the paper was found this time not to have been the least burnt. Lord Lindsay further declares—and as one of the few noblemen who do real scientific work, his evidence must be of some value—that on eight occasions he has had hot coals placed on his own hand by Home without injury. Mr. W. H. Harrison (*Spiritualist*, March, 15, 1870,) saw him take a large coal which covered the palm of his hand and stood six or seven inches high. As he walked about the room it threw a ruddy glow on the walls, and when he came to the table with it, the heat was felt in the faces of all present. The coal was thus held for five minutes. These phenomena have now happened scores of times in the presence of scores of witnesses. They are facts of the reality of which there can be no doubt; and they are altogether inexplicable by the known laws of physiology and heat."

How far these powers are "altogether inexplicable by the known laws of physiology and heat" I propose now briefly to inquire.

There are three ways in which deception may have taken place:

1st. The spectators may have labored under hallucination and delusion.

2d. Mr. Home may have appeared to make use of live coals in his experiments when in reality he did not.

3d. He may have protected his hands, clothing, and Mr. Hall's head by some one or more of the methods at present well known.

1. Although it is by no means impossible that the principle of suggestion or expectant attention may have caused those present simultaneously to imagine that Mr. Home performed all the various acts attributed to him, it is nevertheless much more probable that the true explanation is to be found under one or both of the other heads. At the same time the reader ought clearly to understand that with our present experience of the effects of extreme heat, such as that of a live coal on the human body and ordinary clothing, the weight of evidence is greatly in favor of the postulate that half a dozen people would be more likely to be deceived, than that a man should without protection of any kind, hold live coals in his hand, and put them into his waistcoat pocket, without either being burnt. When in addition, we consider that these people were accustomed to be moved by suggestion and expectant attention, and that the light of the room was dim, the probability is greatly increased. And it is rendered still more predominant when we call to mind the fact that at least two of them (Lord Lindsay and Lord Adare) have since then shown their capacity to be thus deceived, as in the matter of Mr. Home's levitation to which reference has already been made.

As previously stated, the fact that several persons are simultaneously deceived and caused to believe the reality of hallucinations or illusions is common enough. At the very time of writing these lines, the following account appears in the Baltimore *Sun* of February 21st, 1876:—

"The neighborhood of Charles and Mulberry streets was the scene of great excitement on Saturday night over the rumor that there was a burglar in the grocery store of Thomas Reese & Son. Shortly after Mr. Reese had locked the doors and left for home, a citizen in passing was certain that he saw through the plate glass a man moving about in the store, and he got a boy to watch the place until the police could be found. When the policeman arrived, the presence of somebody was confirmed by the boy, who said he saw a man peeping at him from inside the store. A telegraph messenger was dispatched to Mr. Reese to inform him of the circumstances and to get the keys. In the absence of the messenger, a large crowd assembled in front of the store, at least half of whom distinctly saw the burglar moving about the store, and by the time Mr. Reese's two sons arrived with the keys, excitement had reached its highest tension, and the prospect of having a good look at a live burglar was largely speculated upon. The doors were opened and Capt. Jamison, the two sons of Mr. Reese, and two policemen cautiously entered, leaving two policemen to guard the door. The gas was turned on and a careful search made behind boxes, barrels, and bags. Every nook and cranny big enough to hide a rat was closely inspected, but without finding any burglar. The supposed burglar was an optical delusion, caused by the reflection from the lights in a drug store on the opposite side of the street, which gave the inside of Mr. Reese's store the appearance of being lighted up, and the figures seen were the reflection of passers by on the opposite sidewalk."

2d. It would have been a very easy matter for Mr. Home to have caused his company to imagine that he was using real live coals when in fact he was doing nothing of the kind. A good juggler, such as Mr. Home evidently is, would have experienced no difficulty in changing real coals for false ones, so as to give the sensation of heat or cold as desired.

It is well known that a piece of spongy platinum becomes incandescent where a current of hydrogen is allowed to impinge upon it, and that the incandescence is immediately lost when the current of gas is arrested. It is much more reasonable to suppose that Mr. Home employed this substance and a small reservoir of hydrogen, than that he really did, at will or through the will of a spirit, cause a coal of fire to lose and regain its heat.

3d. The means which Mr. Home most probably used are those which are well known to render the skin and clothing more or less incombustible. The repeated application of sulphuric acid to the skin of the hand will enable it to resist the heat of a burning coal for a considerable period, and oil, if rubbed in frequently and for a long time, renders the skin hard and horny. Long, continual exposure of the skin to great heat has also the same effect, as in the case of the copper smelters referred to by Beckmann. According to some authorities, the juice of certain plants produces a like condition when applied to the skin.

It would have been very easy for Mr. Home to place a layer of asbestos cloth under the burning coals laid on Mr. Hall's head and Lord Lindsay's hand, and thus to have effectually prevented injury to the skin. It would have been still easier for him to have thus protected his own hand. In any one of the cases detection would not have been probable, for the attention of the subject and observers being otherwise engaged, deception would have been the natural consequence, just as it is with the dupe out of whose hand the skilful conjurer removes a coin which the victim believes is still firmly grasped. Mr. Home could, with the greatest facility, and with the slightest possible risk of discovery in the badly lighted room, have worn gloves made of asbestos or amianthus cloth. Gloves made of this latter material, according to the method of M. Aldini, enable the wearer to handle red hot coals or iron with impunity. A fireman, having his hand within a double asbestos glove, and his palm protected by a piece of asbestos cloth, seized with impunity a large piece of red hot iron, carried it deliberately to the distance of 150 feet, inflamed straw with it, and brought it back again to the furnace. On other occasions this fireman handled blazing wood and burning substances, and walked during five minutes upon an iron grating placed over flaming faggots.

In the experiments which were made at Paris in the presence of a committee of the Academy of Sciences, two parallel rows of straw and brushwood, supported by iron wires, were erected at a distance of three feet from each other and were thirty feet each in length. When ignited, the heat was so great that it was necessary for the spectators to stand at the distance of eight or ten yards to avoid suffering. The flames from these burning masses seemed to fill up the whole space between them, and rose to the height of nine or ten feet. Then six firemen, clothed in the incombustible dresses, and walking at a slow pace behind each other, repeatedly passed through the whole length between the burning walls, the fire of which was kept up with additional fuel. One of the firemen carried on his back a child eight years old, in a wicker basket covered with wire gauze, and the child had no other dress than a cap made of amianthus cloth.*

Mr. Home's waistcoat pocket, into which he is said to have put a coal of fire, was probably lined with amianthus cloth or made of material rendered incombustible by having been saturated with a solution of alum in water.

Any one of the explanations proposed is infinitely more probable than that Mr. Home did, without protection or previous preparation, carry live coals in his hand and waistcoat pocket, and put them on other people's bodies without causing injury. The latter is an impossibility, so far as our knowledge of the physical effect of heat now extends, and to set aside that knowledge, based as it is on the experience of ages, merely because half a dozen people with badly trained minds think they were witnesses of the alleged phenomena, would be in the highest degree illogical and absurd.

When not thus protected Mr. Home would doubtless suffer as did the devil-possessed priest who presumed too much upon the power of the demon he worshipped, and the account of which is thus given by Mr. Robert Charles Caldwell: †

"But evening draws near; the sunset reddens over the Ghauts; the deep mellow notes of the wood pigeons grow fainter and then cease; fire-flies twinkle out; great bats flap by lazily overhead; then comes the dull tuck of the tom-tom; the fire before the rustic devil-temple is lit; the crowd gathers and

* For the details of these and other experiments of a similar character the reader is referred to Sir David Brewster's Letters on Natural Magic, Letter XII.

† Demonaltry, Devil Dancing, and Demoniacal Possession. *The Contemporary Review.* February, 1876.

waits for the priest. He is there! His lethargy has been thrown aside; the laugh of a fiend is in his mouth. He stands before the people the oracle of the demon, the devil-possessed! Enough for the present. I must subsequently describe this scene more carefully in detail. Suffice it in this place to say that about eight years ago I was staying in Tinnevelly not ten miles distant from the scene of a tragedy on one occasion such as I have referred to. The priest appeared suddenly at the devil-temple before the expectant votaries. A cauldron was over the fire and in it was lead in a molten state. 'Behold' calmly cried the priest, the 'demon is in me, I will prove to you all the presence within me of the omnipotent divinity.' With that he lifted the cauldron and poured the liquid lead over his head. Horns were blown, toms-toms beaten, fresh logs of resinous wood flung into the fire, and goats duly sacrificed. The priest staggered about a little and then fell down in a fainting fit. Three days afterwards he died in horrible agony. But his mind was calm and clear to the last The last words he uttered were *nânê sattaya sâmi!* 'It is indeed I who am the true God.'"

After these supreme performances of Mr. Home it is scarcely necessary to consider those of less moment, such as moving bells and other articles, table-lifting, accordeon-playing, etc. There is only one other which has acquired some importance from having been elaborately studied and then endorsed by Mr. Crookes, and that is the *variation produced in the weights of bodies* by spiritual agency, or, as Mr. Crookes assumes, by a new force which he calls "psychic."

For the determination of the point involved, Mr. Crookes*

* An Experimental Investigation of a New Force. *Quarterly Journal of Science*, July, 1871.

constructed an apparatus consisting of a mahogany board 36 inches long by 9½ inches wide and 1 inch thick. At one end a strip of mahogany was screwed on, forming a foot, the length of which equalled the width of the board. This end of the board rested on a table, while the other end was supported by a spring balance attached to a firm tripod stand. The whole arrangement is shown in the accompanying wood-cut (Fig. 1):

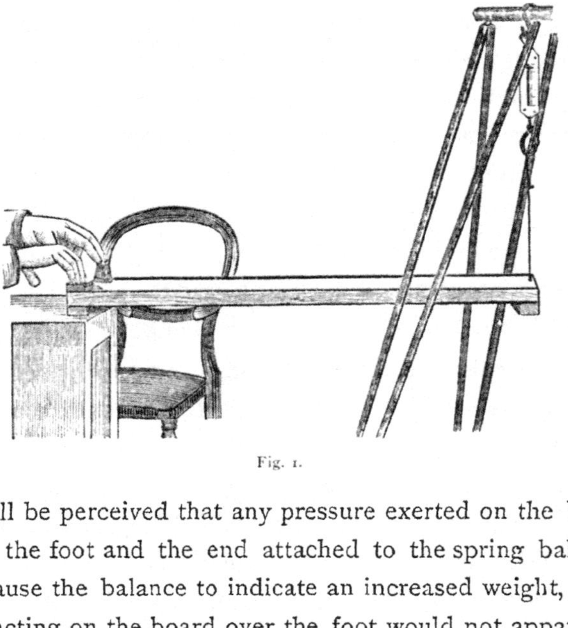

Fig. 1.

It will be perceived that any pressure exerted on the board between the foot and the end attached to the spring balance, would cause the balance to indicate an increased weight, while a force acting on the board over the foot would not apparently affect the balance, and one exerted on the board at its extreme end over the table would cause the other end of the board to rise or would show diminished weight by the indicator of the balance.

Everything being thus arranged, Mr. Home placed the tips of his fingers lightly on the end of the board which was resting on the support, and almost immediately the pointer of the balance was seen to descend. After a few seconds it rose again. This movement was repeated several times.

"Mr. Home now of his own accord took a small hand-bell and a little card match-box which happened to be near, and placed one under each hand, to satisfy us, as he said, that he was not producing the downward pressure. The very slow oscillation of the spring balance became more marked, and Dr. A. B., on watching the index, said that he saw it descend to 6½ lbs. The normal weight of the board as so suspended being 3 lbs. the additional downward pull was therefore 3½ lbs. On looking immediately afterwards at the automatic register we saw that the index had at one time descended as low as 9 lbs., showing a maximum pull of 6 lbs."

In order to see how the indicator would be affected by weight applied to the end of the board resting on the table, Mr. Crookes stepped upon the table and stood on one foot on the end of the board. Dr. A. B., who was observing the index, said that it only indicated an increased weight of 1½ lbs. Mr Crookes' weight was 140 lbs. It is probable that his foot projected slightly over the foot of the board, for otherwise it is very evident the index would not have been depressed.

Mr. Crookes kept full notes of these experiments, afterwards writing them out, and sent the proof of his paper to Dr. Huggins, the eminent astronomer (the Dr. A. B. mentioned), and received from him the following note:

"Upper Tulse Hill, S. W., June 9, 1871.

"Dear Mr. Crookes,—Your proof appears to me to contain a correct statement of what took place in my presence at your house. My position at the table did not permit me to be a witness to the withdrawal of Mr. Home's hand from the accordeon, but such was stated to be the case at the time by yourself and by the person sitting on the other side of Mr. Home.

"The experiments appear to me to show the importance of further investigation, but I wish it to be understood that I express no opinion as to the cause of the phenomena which took place.

"Yours very truly,

"WILLIAM HUGGINS."

"William Crookes, Esq., F. R. S."

Subsequently, Mr. Crookes performed another series of experiments in which additional precautions were taken to avoid error in the conclusions. The apparatus used is thus described.*

"To do away with the objection that the contact of the hand of the medium with the lever in his spring balance experiment, might by some inexplicable possibility produce the observed results by muscular action he tried the following experiment. Over the centre of the fulcrum he placed a glass vessel full of water, and by means of an iron stand quite detached from all the rest of the apparatus, a vessel of copper was held so that it dipped into the water without touching the sides of the glass vessel, the bottom of the copper vessel was perforated with holes in consequence of which it was partially filled with water. The cut on page 105 shows the whole arrangement. (Fig. 2).

"When Mr. Home placed his hands inside the copper vessel, any force passing through his hands had to traverse the water, hence no muscular action of his could have any effect upon the spring balance. With the apparatus thus arranged,

* "Further Experiments of Mr. Crookes," *Spiritual Magazine*, August 1, 1871.

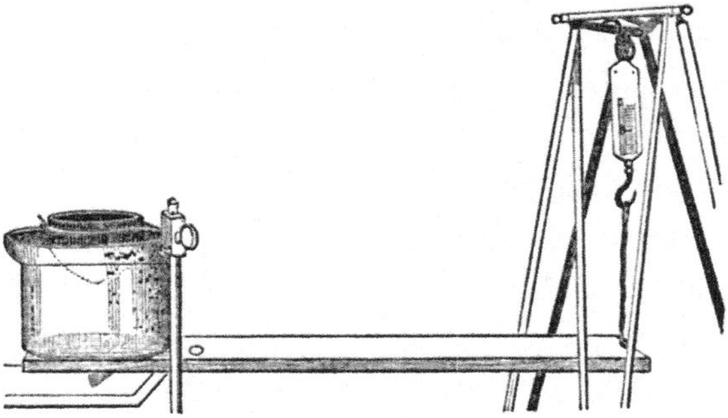

Fig. 2.

the lever oscillated as in his previous experiment, the average strain registered being three or four pounds."

The lever moved equally well when Mr. Home put his hands on the table without touching the apparatus at all.

I think after an attentive consideration of these experiments we may conclude that in point of fact they are correct. There is such a thing as being unduly sceptical as well as weakly credulous, and we should have to strain our scepticism—which is only healthy when it is rational—to an unwarrantable extent were we to disregard the results reported by so accurate an observer as Mr. Crookes, and witnessed and concurred in—so far as the facts go—by so eminent and cautious a philosopher as Mr. Huggins. It is therefore, I think, fairly to be believed that Mr. Home was capable without the exertion of muscular force of so acting on the spring balance through the medium of the board as to indicate an increase of weight.

Increasing and diminishing the weight of bodies are performances well known to the East Indian Jugglers, and their feats in this direction far exceed thand of Mr. Hôme and other so called mediums, if we are to credit the accounts which are given us by observers. Among others, and the most recent is M. Louis Jacolliot,* who is, moreover, sufficiently impressionable, as his work shows, to be readily acted upon by the principle of suggestion. He says.

"I had often seen charmers cause certain objects to adhere to the ground,—either according to the explanation given me by an English Major who had studied the subject, by charging them with a fluid, so as to increase their specific weight or by some other unknown means. I resolved to repeat the experiment. Taking then a little table made of teak-wood that I lifted readily with the thumb and fore finger, I placed it on the terrace and asked the fakir if he could not so fix it in that situation that it would be impossible for me to move it.

"The Malabarian went to the little piece of furniture and placing his hands on the upper surface remained immovable in that position for nearly a quarter of an hour; when this time had elapsed he turned towards me and said, smiling:

"'The spirits have come and no one can displace that table without their consent.' I approached it with a certain amount of incredulity and seizing it made what I thought was the necessary effort to raise it; I could budge it no more than if it had been fastened into the cement of the terrace. I redoubled my efforts and the top of the table came off in my hands. I then vigorously took hold of the legs which remained erect united by two cross pieces but I obtained no other result. At this moment a thought struck me, 'if,' I said to myself,' 'it is by charging objects with a fluid that the

* "Le spiritisme dans le monde. L'initiation et les sciences occultes dans l'Inde." Paris, 1875, p. 294, *et seq.*

charmers produce this effect, and if the phenomenon is only the development of a natural force of which we do not know the cause, the fluid when not renewed by the imposition of the hands of the operator will gradually be lost, and in that case I ought to be able in a few moments to displace what remains of the table.' I then requested the fakir to go to the opposite end of the terrace which he did very willingly, and in the course of a few minutes the little table was readily dislodged from its position.

" 'The *pitris* [spirits] are gone,' said the Hindoo, in explanation of the circumstance, 'because the bond which attached them to the earth has been broken.' "

Now this experiment is not like those of Mr. Crookes, but it appears at first sight similar, and even more astonishing. Like Mr. Home, the fakir attributed the immobility and increased weight of the table to the influence of spirits, but the explanation is quite surely to be found by another line of investigation. M. Jacolliot, by his own account, was subject to vertigo and semi-unconsciousness at times when the fakir was performing some of his more astonishing tricks. The whole scene, as he describes it, may, therefore, have been an illusion or hallucination. The fakir may himself have broken the table or the entire account may be pure imagination.

In this connection, the following story, related of Sir Walter Raleigh,* is apposite.

Sir Walter was in his prison composing the second volume of his history of the world. Leaning on the window sill,

* Quoted by Mr. S. Baring Gould, in "Curious Myths of the Middle Ages." London, 1869, p. 114.

he was thinking of the work before him, when suddenly his attention was attracted by a loud noise in the court yard, upon which his cell looked. He saw one man strike another whom he supposed by his dress, to be an officer. The latter immediately drawing his sword, ran his assailant through the body. The wounded man then knocked the officer down with a stick, and fell dead upon the pavement. At this moment the guard arrived, first carried off the officer in an insensible condition, and then removed the corpse of the man who had been run through the body. The following day Raleigh was visited by a friend to whom he related the event of the day before which had occurred under his eyes. To his astonishment his friend unhesitatingly declared that Sir Walter had entirely mistaken the whole series of incidents.

The supposed officer was no officer at all, but the servant of a foreign ambassador; it was he who had dealt the first blow; he had not drawn his sword, but the other had snatched it from his side, and had run *him* through the body before any one could interfere; whereupon a stranger from among the crowd knocked the murderer down with his stick and some of the foreigners belonging to the ambassador's retinue, carried off the corpse. The friend of Raleigh added that government had ordered the arrest and immediate trial of the murderer as the man assassinated was one of the principal servants of the Spanish ambassador.

"Excuse me," said Raleigh, "but I cannot have been deceived, as you supposed, for I was eye-witness to the events which took place under my own window, and the man fell on that spot where you see a paving stone standing up above the rest." "My dear Raleigh," replied his friend, "I was sitting on that stone, when the fray took place, and I received this scratch on my cheek in snatching the sword from the murderer, and upon my word of honor, you have been deceived in every particular."

Sir Walter, when alone, took up the second volume of his history, which was in MS., and contemplating it, thought, "If I cannot believe my own eyes, how can I be assured of the truth of a tithe of the events which happened ages before I was born?" and he flung the manuscript into the fire.

But we may admit that the circumstances detailed by Jacolliot really occurred, and still we have a better explanation either than that of spiritual influence or a new force, the laws of which have not been studied. For instance, I find in a recently issued book by Mr. J. Stanley Grimes * some personal experiences which are in all respects as reliable as those detailed by Mr Crookes and M. Jacolliot. Mr. Grimes is a lecturer on phrenology, animal magnetism, electro-biology, etc. He expresses the utmost contempt for spiritualistic doctrines, and attributes the performances of mediums either to downright fraud or to some one of the semi-abnormal conditions with which educated physicians are well acquainted. Thus he says:

"We are now prepared to understand another class of experiments to which I have not before alluded. Say to the subject, 'You cannot put your hat on.' He takes the hat and tries to put it on, but his hand moves the hat to one side and then to the other side, but will not obey his will. He seems to make great efforts, and nearly succeeds and then repeats his

* "Mysteries of the Head and the Heart explained," etc. Chicago, 1875, p. 285.

efforts, but in vain. Tell him that he cannot sit down, or get up, or open his eyes, or speak, and he tries and fails in the same manner. The modern spiritualists and some others assert that there are two wills contending; that one is the will of the operator and the other that of the subject; but it is easy to prove that this is not true. Any one who will perform the experiment will find that the mere unexpressed will of the operator is ineffectual. The truth is that both the contending forces are in the brain of the subject himself—one force is his own proper and normal will and this is rendered abortive by the superior force of the conforming faculties.

"In Judge Edmonds' book on spiritualism, he gives an account of a performance with a table, which several men could not hold still. In spite of their efforts, the spirits pushed it over and held it down till the spirits were requested to allow it to be raised, when it was lifted with great ease. In this case one force was supposed to be the wills of the men who had hold of the table, and the other force to be exerted by some invisible spirit. In reality both forces resided in the brains of the distinguished operators themselves.

"I often perform an experiment involving the same principles in the presence of large audiences. After a person is found to be susceptible and conforming, I ask him to take hold of a table and hold it still if he can. I then ask the spirit to push it over towards him. He will take hold of the table and while he seems to be holding it up, an unseen power appears to be pushing it over. He is in reality holding it up with one hand and pulling it over with the other. If his conforming organs are sufficiently excited the experiment will succeed perfectly; the table will go over and he will be unable to raise it again until I request the spirit to allow him to do so."

"I usually call on the spirit of Sampson to push the table over and at the same time urge the young man, the subject, to hold it up. If the audience are unacquainted with mesmerism and inclined to believe in spiritualism, they generally regard me as a wonderful medium and suppose that a spirit is really moving the table. To give greater effect to the performance I use encouraging language to both parties. I say push young man! push spirit! push both of you! Sometimes I have two or three subjects take hold of the table and in trying to hold it they occasionally demolish it."

But I have recently performed an experiment similar in all essential results to that reported by M. Jacolliot. I took a small oblong Japanese table weighing only a pound and a half, and in the presence of a young man of a highly impressionable nervous organization, and hence peculiarly well fitted to be acted upon by the force of suggestion, placed it upon the floor of my consulting-room, raising a corner of the rug so that it could rest upon the bare floor. I then said to him, "I am going to make this table so heavy that you cannot raise it, please give me your attention for a few minutes."

I then placed the ends of my fingers of both hands on the table and stood in that position for about fifteen minutes. During this procedure, the young man looked at the table and me with the greatest interest, and when I saw from the expression of his face that his attention was sufficiently concentrated, I removed my hands and told him the table was now fastened to the floor, and that he could not lift it. He took hold of the light object with both hands, and appeared to be making strong efforts to raise it from the floor, but he could not, and I saw that so far from endeavoring to lift it as he supposed he was doing, he was in reality pressing it with all his might towards the floor. Finally he broke the top of the table in half, not by holding, but by pushing. He then desisted from his exertions and asked me to lighten the table so that he could lift it. I made a few passes over it, and then telling him he could raise it easily, he took hold of it and succeeded of course, without any appreciable exertion.

Now I am unable to perceive in what respect this experiment differs from that detailed by M. Jacolliot, and I think the reader will require no suggestion to enable him to appreciate the fact that in both cases it was not the apparent but the real performer, M. Jacolliot, in the one instance, and my impressionable subject in the other, who kept the table from moving. In both cases the individuals who attempted to raise the tables were so impressed by one overwhelming idea that they could not, that their actions were unconsciously directed in accordance therewith. That this principle of suggestion and its influence are competent to explain many of the phenomena of spiritualism has already been insisted on, and need not, therefore, further detain us. We may, therefore, pass at once to the consideration of Mr. Crookes' experiments.

We would scarcely be entirely justified in applying the principle of suggestion to the phenomena alleged to have taken place through Mr. Home, and in presence of Messrs. Crookes and Huggins. These two gentlemen are not of the class of individuals in which "subjects" are included, and the precautions taken to avoid error and the numerous checks devised to ensure exactness preclude the idea of any mistake so far as the facts are concerned. It may, therefore, be assumed with as much certainty as we can ever have in regard to any event, that when Mr. Home placed his hands on the apparatus in the manner described, the index of the spring balance descended. There is only one other alternative, and that is, that Mr. Crookes and Mr. Home were in a conspiracy together to deceive Dr. Huggins. No one acquainted with Mr. Crookes' character, devotion to science and truth, and position in society, could for one moment adopt that explanation. It may be added too, that Dr. Huggins is a gentleman whose whole life has been passed with apparatus and instruments, whose mind is pre-eminent for its scientific training, and that consequently his liability to be deceived is exceedingly small.

But in admitting the facts, we go as far as it is possible to advance without meeting with uncertainties and assumptions. To attribute the falling of the index of the spring balance to spiritual agency is about as sensible as to allege its causation by lunar influence. Indeed, far less so, for we know that the moon does exert a very powerful effect upon the earth, and we have no satisfactory evidence to show that spiritual beings affect in any way the substances belonging to our planet or even that such beings exist. Neither is Mr. Crookes much more happy with his "psychic force." Because a spring balance with a board attached to it indicates increased weight when a person touches the arrangement in the manner described, is certainly no adequate reason for rushing to the conclusion that a new force has been discovered. Mr. Huggins, while admitting the facts, exercises a proper degree of philosophical caution when he declines to express an opinion relative to the cause of the phenomenon. There are so many ways in which known forces manifest themselves and so little is known of the laws which govern them, that Mr. Crookes might, for the present, with safety and propriety, have held his opinion in abeyance. Of course such a thing as a "psychic force" is possible. But possibilities and actualities are very different things, and it will require much more evidence than that now submitted to remove Mr. Crookes' new power from the one category to the other.

But the best evidence against the existence of spiritualistic force in the matter of Mr. Crookes' experiment, is the fact that the index can be made to move in the way and probably to the extent mentioned by him by similar pressure exerted by many persons not pretenders to mediumistic powers, and in whom there is no evidence tending to show the existence of any hitherto unknown force.

An inspection of the apparatus (Fig. 1) will show that if a downward tractile force be exerted on the board at any point in front of the foot, at the end which rests upon the table, the extremity attached to the spring balance will be depressed and the index will consequently show increased weight.

An experiment recently described by Prof. Tyndall * illustrates this fact very clearly.

Place an egg in an egg-cup and balance a long lath upon the egg as shown in Fig. 3, on opposite page.

Though the lath be almost a plank it will obediently follow a rod of glass, gutta-percha or sealing-wax, which has been previously well dried and rubbed, the former with a piece of silk, and the two latter with woollen cloth.

* Lessons in Electricity; Holiday Lectures at the Royal Institution; *Popular Science Monthly*, March, 1876, p. 611.

Now in dry weather, many persons within my knowledge, have only to walk with a shuffling gait over the carpet, and then approaching the lath hold out the finger instead of the glass, sealing-wax or gutta-percha, and instantly the end of the lath

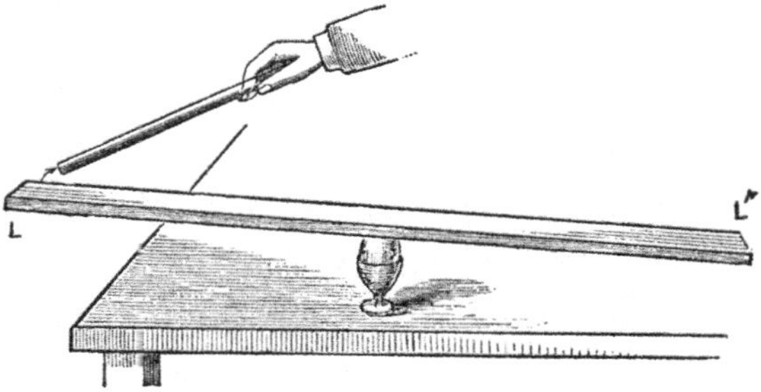

Fig. 3.

at L rises to meet it, and the end at L' is depressed. Applying these principles, I arranged an apparatus exactly like that of Prof. Crookes, except that the spring balance was such as is used for weighing letters and was therefore very delicate, indicating quarter-ounces with exactness, and that the board was thin and narrow.

Applying the glass rod or stick of sealing wax to the end resting by its foot on the table, the index of the balance at once descended, showing an increased weight of a little over three quarters of an ounce, and this without the board being raised from the table.

I then walked over a thick Turkey rug for a few moments, and holding my finger under the board near the end attached to the balance, caused a fall of the index of almost half an ounce. I then rested my finger lightly on the end of the board immediately over the foot, and again the index descended and oscillated several times just as in Mr. Home's experiments. The lowest point reached was six and a quarter ounces, and as the board weighed, as attached to the balance, five ounces, there was an increased weight of one and a quarter ounces. At no time was the end of the board raised from the table.

I then arranged the apparatus so as to place a thin glass tumbler nearly full of water immediately over the fulcrum as in Mr. Crookes' experiment (Fig. 2), and again the index fell and oscillated on my fingers being put into the water.

Now if one person can thus, with a delicate apparatus like mine, cause the index, through electricity, to descend and ascend, it is not improbable that others, like Mr. Home, could show greater, or even different, electrical power, as in Mr. Crookes' experiments. It is well known that all persons are not alike in their ability to be electrically excited. Many persons, myself among them, can light the gas with the end of the finger. Others cannot do it with any amount of shuffling over the carpet. At any rate is it not much more probable that Mr. Home's experiments are to be thus explained than by attributing the results to spiritualism or psychic force?

As to the other manifestations mentioned by Mr. Crookes, such as playing on the accordeon, they are doubtless, if real, to be explained in like manner to those with the spring balance.

The balls of fire which are reported as among the phenomena attendant on mediumistic influence scarcely require consideration here; recalling to mind that if they were really perceived, it is highly illogical and unscientific to attribute them to spiritual agency, when our knowledge of electricity tells us that just such balls are not at all uncommon in certain electrical conditions of the atmosphere.

It is, however by no means certain that these globes of fire were actually perceived by the persons who so report. Appearances such as these are not infrequent among the symptoms of cerebral congestion, and ocular disease. Most physicians having met with cases of the kind.

As to the other alleged spiritualistic performance of physical mediums, such as the so called materialization of the body —Katie King, etc.—the ringing of bells, getting loose from cords and bands, moving of tables, knockings, and many other juggling tricks of similar character, they are to be regarded in the light of what has already been said, and time would be wasted in taking them up and dealing with them separately.

CHAPTER VII.

SENSITIVE OR IMPRESSIBLE MEDIUMS.

A SENSITIVE or impressible medium is, according to Kardec, one who feels the presence of spirits by a vague im pression, a kind of light touch on the surface of the body, which cannot be explained by reference to ordinary causes.

Here the evidence—if such it can be called—is entirely subjective; a sensation, the existence of which, is only realized by the subject. That many mediums feel impressions such as those mentioned is very probably true. All the various forms of numbness, such as tingling, formication, a sensation such as if water were trickling over the skin, pins and needles sticking in it, or as if the part were "asleep," are common enough among the people from whom mediums are constituted. Such phenomena are merely symptoms of nervous derangement of some kind, often slight in character, but not infrequently of serious moment. In the former case they may generally be dissipated by a few doses of the bromide of potassium or half a dozen applications of galvanism; in the latter, they are often precursors of organic disturbance of the brain or spinal cord, leading to paralysis, epilepsy or mental derangement.

A lady not long since was under my care who imagined that

she could discern the presence of a spirit by a sensation of coldness which extended throughout one side of her body, and which was paroxysmal in character. She was brought to me by her husband, a gentleman of good sense and education, very much against her will, and refused persistently to be subjected to medical treatment. A few days afterwards she had a cerebral hemorrhage, and was deprived of both the power of motion and of sensibility in the very parts in which she had experienced the spiritual manifestations. She was cured of her delusion, but at rather a heavy price. Such erroneous conceptions of the nature of sensations, the physiology of which is thoroughly understood, have existed at all times of the world's history, and even at the present day form part of the religious system of certain barbarous and semi-barbarous nations. It is well known to us all that under the influence of intense emotional disturbance we experience feelings which are of the same character, in fact, identical with those which M. Kardec tells us are produced by contact with a spirit. Thus we thrill with pleasure and delight on hearing a melodious or harmonious piece of music, or with admiration or sympathy for the bearing or misfortunes of the characters which interest us in a play; we tingle with shame or anger, our fingers itch to get at an enemy, and an electric shudder goes through us when we are struck with horror.

Similar sensations are even excited through the other senses in the first place, and by mere force of imagination thereafter. Herbert Spencer says "I cannot think of seeing a slate rubbed with a dry sponge without there running through me the same thrill that actually seeing it produces." I have already considered the effects produced upon various parts of the body by con centrated attention; undoubtedly, most of the "vague impressions" and sensations of "light touches" which, according to M. Kardec, indicate the presence of spirits, are to be ascribed to this factor.

CHAPTER VIII.

SEEING AND AUDITIVE MEDIUMS.

SEEING and auditive mediums are those who, according to our authority Kardec, are capable of seeing and hearing spirits ; in other words, they see apparitions and hear voices. Medical science teaches us that such hallucinations are very common even in persons not the subjects of insanity. I have already in the early part of this work considered this division of the subject so far as relates to furnishing a satisfactory explanation of the causes of erroneous sensorial impressions, especially of those of sight and hearing. It is extremely probable, however, that so far as the so called mediums are concerned, the stories which they tell in regard to seeing spirits and hearing their conversation are pure fabrications. It may be laid down as a law admitting of no exception that, *cæteris paribus*, one individual is just as capable of seeing a spirit and hearing its voice as another. When therefore, several persons are assembled together under like circumstances, and one of them asserts that he or she sees a spirit which the others do not see, either the person making the declaration labors under hallucination, or utters a falsehood. Even if all the others were to declare they saw a spirit, the evidence still would not be convincing till we had carefully inquired into all the circumstances, intrin-

6

sic and extrinsic, of the individuals. For it is infinitely more probable that half a dozen or more persons should be mistaken in regard to an event so thoroughly at variance with the experience of mankind than that they should really have seen a spirit.

And the mistake may arise from a like cause acting simultaneously on a number of persons and producing like results as in the examples previously cited ; or deception may be practised by designing persons and the apparent spirit may be real flesh and blood as in the Katie King case, so thoroughly exposed in Philadelphia a year ago ; or by means of mirrors and lenses, and a slight knowledge of the laws of optics, the image of a real person may be made to project in such a manner as to convey the idea of an incorporeal being, as in Prof. Pepper's ghost so often brought into use now in theatrical performances, and in Benvenuto Cellini's demons in the Coliseum.

In a recent work of Mr. Robert Dale Owen,* he gives an example in which an apparition was seen by himself and others which has been the means of perverting several very excellent people within my knowledge into the vagaries of spiritualism, and of shaking the confidence of others endowed with somewhat more of intellectual force. No one who knows him will question Mr. Owen's honesty, especially after his recantation in regard to the Katie King fraud. But Mr. Owen has never to my knowledge retracted his assertions relative to the apparition referred to, and in order that the readers of this volume may perceive upon what flimsy evidence an example rests which Mr. Owen refers to as constituting an era in his spiritual experience, and

* "The Debatable Land between this World and the Next." New York, 1872, p. 472, *et seq.*

to show in what way the appearance was in all probability produced, I quote his account in full.

"What I particularly desired was to have an opportunity, in the light, of witnessing the formation of such an apparition; its actions, its movements from place to place, and its disappearance. But it was not until the year 1867 that I obtained any further satisfaction. During the spring of that year I heard of Miss B——, of Boston, an elderly lady long known and esteemed in that city, as a successful teacher of music and dancing. It was said that she, in a private circle, had obtained numerous objective apparitions in a partially lighted room. This was afterwards confirmed to me by a most estimable lady who had herself been present at many of those sittings; Mrs. John Davis, widow of the well known ex-governor of Massachusetts, and of whom I have already spoken.

"Mrs. Davis expressed to me her conviction that Miss B—— was entirely sincere and disinterested; and that the phenomena which she (Mrs. Davis) had witnessed in Miss B——'s apartments were genuine. Miss B——, it seems, had several friends, married ladies in the middle rank of life, who had more or less power as mediums, especially in connection with spiritual appearances of an objective character. On several occasions, sometimes in one of their houses, sometimes in another, Miss B—— had herself seen an apparition.

"None of those ladies were professional mediums; but it occurred to them that if they met occasionally they might by their united powers obtain very interesting results. Miss B—— offered the use of her spacious apartments; and during a series of experiments which were conducted there, phenomena of a marvellous character were observed; a great variety of spirits appearing, chiefly strangers to any of the assistants, in various costumes.

"This was noised abroad and brought requests from the curious for admission to witness such wonders. These were usually granted, but uniformly as a favor and without charge. Opinions were various; some visitors were convinced, others went away in doubt whether it was not an exhibition got up to mystify the credulous or gratify a longing for notoriety.

"This of course was very unpleasant to the ladies concerned, and when I called on Miss B—— in May, 1867, I found that for several months they had almost ceased to meet. When, however, I expressed to Miss B—— my earnest desire to investigate the matter, intending some day to publish the results, she acceded to my wishes with the utmost alacrity. 'I am so glad' she said 'to have some one who will be listened to, to test these phenomena. When one has no other interest or desire than to get at an important truth, it seems hard to be subjected to groundless suspicions.'

"At the first two or three sittings a portion only of the ladies could attend, and Miss B—— was of the opinion that the discontinuance of their regular sittings had for the time weakened their power. We had only rapping and phosphorescent phenomena, but of a remarkable character. Bright stars appeared on the person of one medium, and a line of light along the forehead of another, the word 'Hope' on the back of the hand of a third. These appearances were brilliant and could be seen twenty feet off across a dimly lighted room. At other times the raps were so violent as to shake the sofa on which we sat.

"But until the session of June 4th there was no apparition.

On that occasion we had one under very satisfactory circumstances but I did not consider the test complete; for I did not witness either the formation of the figure or its disappearance.

"It was not until the twenty fifth of June that we were able to bring together all the ladies who had composed the original circle. I consider that day, like the twenty-first of October, 1860, an era in my spiritual experience.

"AN APPARITION IN SHINING RAIMENT.

"Miss B——'s rooms, which occupied the entire third floor of a corner house in Washington Street, Boston, consisted of a large apartment thirty feet front by thirty-five feet deep; opening by folding doors into a parlor back of it which was twenty-five feet by twenty. From each room there was one door of exit only, on a passage or stair-landing, as seen in diagram (Fig. 4) on following page.

"The front room was lighted by eight windows, four on Washington Street, and four on a gas-lit court-yard. As there were no curtains drawn nor shutters closed during the sitting, which was held after lamp-lighting, this room was so far lit from without that by any-one seated in the back parlor a few feet from the folding doors, the dress and general appearance of persons in the front room could be readily observed, and every motion they made distinctly seen. I took notice, however, that there was not light enough to recognize features except close at hand. In this room, employed for dancing lessons, the floor was uncarpeted and waxed. All footsteps of persons walking across it could be very distinctly heard."

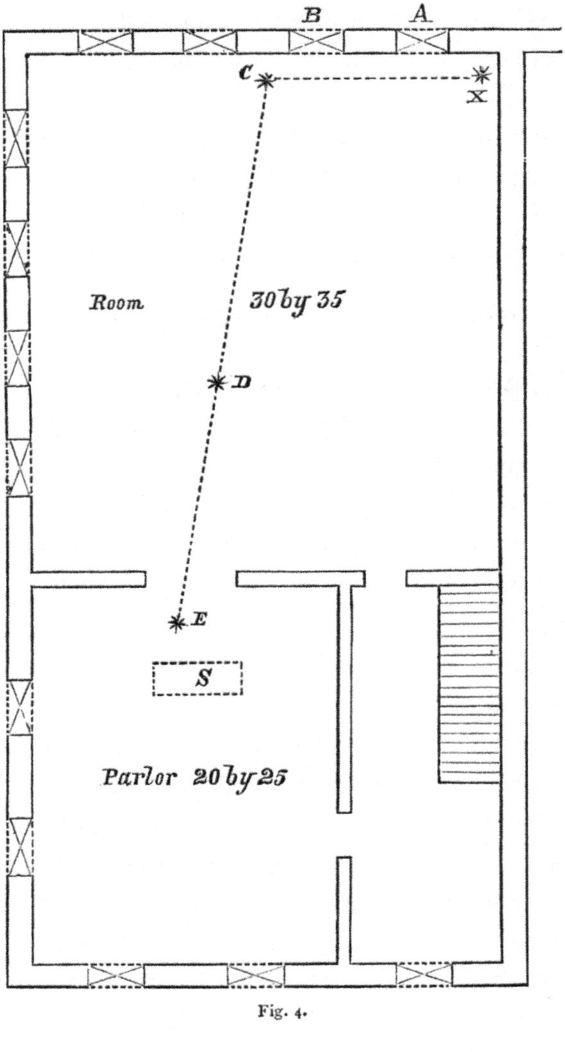

Fig. 4.

"Except myself there was but one visitor present, Mrs. John Davis. The amateur mediums who assisted at the sitting were six in number; Mrs. S. I. D——, Mrs. George N. B——, Mrs. Sarah A. K——, Mrs. Fanny C. P——, Mrs. William H. C——, and Mrs. Mary Ann C——; all ladies, apparently from thirty to forty years of age.

"Before the sitting began, Mrs. Davis and myself passed around the room and examined carefully every part of it. The furniture consisted of a sofa, a piano, and numerous chairs set against the walls. There was no pantry or press or recess of any kind. We locked the sole door of exit and Mrs. Davis kept the key in her pocket during the sitting. Then we locked the door of the back parlor, retaining the key.

"We sat down in that parlor directly before the folding doors. The sofa (marked S on ground plan) on which Mrs. Davis, Miss B—— and myself were seated was about four or five feet within the parlor. I sat on the left hand corner of this sofa; the entrance through the folding doors was draped by curtains which were looped back so that from where I sat I could see three of the four front windows looking out on Washington Street and the corner of the room to the right of them. The six mediums sat three each side of us."

"All was quiet during the early part of the sitting which commenced a little after eight P. M. Scarcely any rapping. A few phosphorescent lights.

"About a quarter past nine, all the mediums being seated by us, I saw dimly, near the right hand corner of the front line of the large room (at X) at first a grayish slightly luminous vapor; after a time a figure draped in white. At first it was stationary; then it moved very slowly past the two right hand windows

(A and B) to the center of the front line of the room (at C) between two windows. There it remained one or two minutes, still but indistinctly visible. Then very slowly, and without sound of footstep, it advanced down the room coming directly toward the center of the folding doors. It stopped (at D) about twelve or fourteen feet from where I was sitting. Thereupon, of a sudden, a brilliant light, coming from the right, striking directly on the figure, and only on it, not directly illuminating the rest of the room—enabled me to see the appearance as perfectly as if the entire room had been lit with gas.

"It was a female figure of medium size, veiled and draped from head to foot in white. The drapery did not resemble in material, anything I had ever seen worn. It gave me, as on a previous occasion, the exact feeling of the scriptural expression 'shining raiment.' Its brilliancy was a good deal like that of new fallen snow in the sunshine; recalling the text which declares the garments of Christ during his transfiguration to have been 'exceeding white as snow;' or again, it was not unlike the purest and freshest Parian marble with a bright light on it, only more brilliant. It had not at all the glitter of spangles or any shining ornament; the tone being as uniform as that of a newly sculptured statue. It stood upright in a graceful attitude, motionless. Had I suddenly seen it elsewhere, and without having witnessed its previous movements I might have imagined it a beautiful piece of sculpture of singularly pure material and marvellously lighted up. The drapery fell around the figure closely, as usual in a statue; not at all according to the modern fashion of amplitude. I think it was shown to us under the bright light as long as fifteen or twenty seconds."

" Mrs. K—— stepped out to meet it, going close up to it, and then returning to us. The figure followed her, and as Mrs. K——, when she passed the folding doors had stepped aside to the right, the apparition advanced with a gliding motion into the parlor till as nearly as I could judge it was within two or three feet of me. Then it stopped (at E).

" As it remained immovable, I raised my left arm hoping to that I should be touched. As I stretched it out, the figure extended its right arm covered with drapery towards me; and dropped into my hand what proved to be a white rose; but its hand did not touch mine.

" Thereupon the appearance, still keeping its face to us, slowly retired with the same silent gliding motion which had marked its advance; not the slighest sound of footstep on the waxed floor being audible.

" A second time it stopped again about twelve or fifteen feet from me, and a second time an instantaneous light coming from the right and falling upon it gave it to be seen with the utmost distinctness. I was enabled to verify my former observation in regard to its appearance, and the unique, rich, resplendent character of the drapery.

" Then it slowly receded, still facing us, to the centre of the opposite wall (at C), gradually diminishing in brightness; and finally it vanished before my eyes.

" Mrs. K—— had followed it, and remained a few seconds near the spot where it vanished. Then I saw her cross the window to the right on her return to us. She was dressed in black.

" I am *quite certain* that one figure only, that of Mrs. K——, as she returned to us, left the spot. From the time the figure in white reached that spot, I kept my eyes intently fixed there *without taking them off for a single moment;* and the light from the street was such that it was impossible for any object, black or white, to pass one of the windows without my seeing it.

"When a minute had elapsed after the disappearance of the figure and while my eyes still fixed on the spot, the thought rushed vividly upon me. 'Is it possible that there can be nothing there?' This thought, *to which I did not give utterance*, had hardly crossed my mind when, as if in reply to it, the same sort of mysterious light which had previously illuminated the figure, suddenly passed the space of wall between the two windows where the figure had disappeared, completely lighting it up —*while the windows and wall on either side were not illuminated.* The light remained long enough to show me that there was nothing whatever there except two chairs set against the wall as I had seen them before the sitting began.

"Then with my eyes still fixed on the place of disappearance I rose and passed entirely around the room; nor did I for a moment take my eyes off the spot that had been illuminated till I had reached it. Everything in the room was exactly as it had been before the sitting, so far as I could recollect. The outer door was still locked.

"It is proper to add that two of the mediums, Mrs. K—— and Mrs. D——, informed me after the sitting was over that they did not remember seeing anything of the figure; both having awoke as from a trance at the close of the sitting. This, Miss B—— informed me, was usual with them.

"I do not think that any of the assistants perceived the formation of the apparition as soon as I did; but while the figure was advancing and retreating, the whispered remarks of the ladies near me—'There it is'—'Now it stops'—'Didn't you see that light?' etc,—made me aware that they saw it just as I did. This was confirmed to me after inquiry by all the ladies except Mrs. K—— and Mrs. D——. All the others observed the sudden illumination of the spot where the figure disappeared.

"As on a former occasion, it is proper I should state here, that throughout the sitting, though the impression produced was profound, solemn beyond expression, never to be forgotten, yet it did not partake at all of the emotion of fear. The predominant feeling was a deep anxiety that there might be no interruption, and that the sitting might not terminate until I had obtained incontrovertible evidence of the fact that the appearance was of a spiritual character, yet as real as any earthly phenomenon.

"The allegation by raps at the close of the sitting was that the apparition was that of Violet. Some years before during a sitting with Kate Fox, I had had a promise, purporting to come from her, that some day when the conditions were favorable she would appear to us. The veil quite concealed the features; but the height, the form, and the carriage of the figure, so strictly corresponded to hers, that when it approached me I ceased to doubt that she had kept her promise."

Now let us analyze this extraordinary account of Mr. Owen's.

1. In the first place, doubt had been thrown upon previous performances at Miss B—'s house and she had been suspected of trickery. If the manifestations which she superintended were real why should they have excited suspicion. If Prof. Dalton, for instance, were to announce a hitherto unknown fact in physiology, we should not suspect him of attempting to commit

a fraud upon the public. There would be no occasion for doubt any more than that being human he might be in error. Miss B——, however, exclaimed that it was "hard to be subjected to groundless suspicion," and the feeling seems to have been so strong against her and her associates that they had actually given up their sittings till in a fortunate moment they came across Mr. Owen, who, as he would be listened to, would unwittingly minister to their thirst for notoriety.

2. An inspection of the diagram of Miss B——'s apartments and attention to the account of the situation which Mr. Owen occupied, will show that it was entirely practicable for any one to have walked along the wall on the right side of the front room without being visible before arriving at the point marked X, the place where the apparition was first perceived by him.

3. The fact that Mr. Owen saw the doors locked and the keys placed in Mrs. Davis' pocket, was no bar to any one else having a key which opened the door leading to the front room from the passage-way at the head of the stairs.

4. A barefooted person walking on the floor would have made no noise.

5. The light was too dim to admit of Mr. Owen distinguishing the features of any such person.

6. He did not touch the hand of the apparition.

7. A dark lantern held at the doorway of the front room opening on the passage-way would have sufficed to illuminate the figure throughout its whole course up to the folding doors, and to have given the flash of light after the disappearance of the apparition. A sudden shutting off of the light would have given the appearance to the figure of vanishing.

8. Mrs. K—— followed the figure. Why did not Mr. Owen follow it and grasp it. If he had he would very certainly have had an earlier experience of the frauds of spiritualists than he had with the Katie King humbug.

The conclusion therefore which every person not willing to be deceived must inevitably arrive at is:—That a confederate woman entered the front room at the doorway leading from the stairs; that she passed noiselessly along the right-hand wall appearing at X; that she was barefooted; that she was illuminated by a dark lantern held at the door or even in the room by another confederate and which came from the right—the only direction from which it could come without Mr. Owen perceiving its source; that she carefully avoided touching Mr. Owen; and that she retired precisely in the same direction in which she had made her appearance.

Mr. Owen was therefore egregiously deceived, and the confederates were Miss B——, Mrs. K——, Mrs. D—— and two others unknown, one of whom played the part of the apparition while the other held the lantern.

As to the object, a desire for notoriety, or to play a practi cal joke, or to accomplish some other desired end would have been a sufficient incentive. Whatever it was it was eminently successful. The conspirators knew how credulous and guileless was the gentleman they selected, or rather who forced himself upon them as their victim, and they took advantage of their opportunity. And this is the sort of evidence upon which the phenomena of spiritualism rests! That full and free inquiry, without which no doctrines in science are at the present day accepted, is expressly forbidden, and inquirers are compelled to remain passive and in the dark while the juggling goes on. That there should be men of intellect weak enough to be deceived by such transparent trickery would be surprising, were it not true that in all ages of the world there have been individuals whose general high intellectual development has not prevented their being made the dupes of designing persons. Such persons lack that power of discrimination between the false and the true, between the probable and improbable, which is sometimes characteristic of the human mind in its very highest phase of expansion. They view facts unequally, as Czermak* forcibly puts it, and thus are ready, in their intense desire to explain anything they do not understand, to adopt a conclusion which is without the least relation with the observed phenomenon.

Take for instance a case the details of which are given by Kardec.†

One evening he was at the opera in company with an excellent "seeing medium." Weber's opera Oberon was being sung, and the medium declared that there were a great many spirits present who occupied the vacant seats and walked through the aisles near the spectators. On the stage another scene was being enacted, for behind the actors were spirits of jovial humor who imitated the gestures of the performers in a grotesque manner, while others of more serious turn seemed to be endeavoring to inspire the singers with additional energy. One spirit was always near one of the principal female singers, and Kardec thought his behavior rather frivolous. After the fall of the curtain this spirit was summoned; he immediately

* Hypnotism in Animals. Lectures delivered at the University of Leipsic. Translated for the *Popular Science Monthly*, Sept. and Nov., 1873, by Clara Hammond.

† *Op. Cit.*, p. 205.

made his appearance in Kardec's box and reproached him with some severity for his hasty judgment. "I am not what you think," said he; "I am her protecting spirit, and I am charged with the duty of guarding her." After a few minutes' serious conversation he departed, saying, "Adieu, she is in her box, and I must go and watch over her."

The spirit of Weber, the author of the opera, was then evoked, and he was asked what he thought of the execution of his work—"It is not very bad," he answered, "but it is too subdued; they sing well, but that is all. There is no inspiration. Wait!" he added, "I will see if I cannot give them a little sacred fire." Then he was seen (by the medium and Kardec) walking about among the singers. A vapor seemed to go out from him and to spread itself over them and from that moment there was a notable increase of energy.

And this is the stuff sensible people are expected to believe, with much more, fully as nonsensical; to some of which, in the performance of the task assumed, I will have to ask the further attention of the reader.

CHAPTER IX.

SPEAKING MEDIUMS.

A SPEAKING medium is one of whom the spirits make use for the purpose of conveying their ideas to the world. It is not therefore in strictness the medium who speaks, but the spirit who animates him. Indeed, the medium is generally in a state of trance, and is not only not aware of the words he is uttering, but may express ideas directly contrary to those he is known to entertain. Even when awake, he rarely preserves the memory of what he has said; he is therefore the mere passive agent under the control of the spirit using him.

Such is the doctrine of the spiritualists. Its absurdity will I think be apparent from the facts I shall adduce in the present connection, and when we come to the consideration of other divisions of the subject.

The hypothesis that individuals could be thus made use of to express the thoughts of spirits of various kinds, good and bad, has been held with more or less pertinacity in all periods of the world's history, has faded out again and again, to be revived under different forms, according to the prevailing superstition of the current time. It is probably less generally held at the present day than at any other, for the reason that there is certainly a growing disposition to disbelieve in matters the affirmation of which cannot be established by proof.

It has even been asserted that the inferior animals could be thus taken possession of, and be employed to give utterance to speeches intended for the edification, reproof or warning of man. Balaam's ass spoke, to go no further back into the recesses of ages, and the fables of Esop were probably based, to some extent at least, upon actual belief.

The oracles of the ancients often spoke through animals. Apis, the sacred bull of the Egyptians, gave his opinion, on being fed by those who consulted him,* and even inanimate objects, as the Sphynx, the statue of Memnon, and the head of Apollo, were at times endowed with the faculty of speech.

In our own day speaking animals are occasionally encountered. Comte, the French conjuror, on one occasion, while travelling near Nevers, overtook a man who was beating his ass. Throwing his voice in the direction of the poor brute's head, Comte upbraided the fellow for his cruelty. The man stared at the ass for a moment in fear and trembling, and then incontinently took to his heels.

At another time, being in the market place at Mâcon, he asked a woman the price of a pig she had for sale, and upon being told, pronounced it exorbitant: a charge which was indignantly denied.

"I will ask the pig," said Comte gravely. "Piggy, is the good woman asking a fair price for you?"

"Too much by half," the pig seemed to reply. "I am measled, and she knows it."

The woman gasped and stared, but she was equal to the occasion.

* Pliny, Hist. Nat., lib. viii., c. 48.

"Oh! the villain!" she exclaimed. "He has bewitched my pig! Police, seize the sorcerer!"

The bystanders rushed to the spot, but Comte slipped away and left the affair to the intelligence of the police.*

This is the only way in which animals, except parrots, ravens and "Ned, the learned seal," are known to speak in our time.

The instances of inspired persons speaking are much more numerous; for the reason probably that the fact of inspiration rests entirely upon the assertion of the speaker. Many cases of the kind are recorded by Görres and other authorities, and cases, before the era of spiritualism, were common in all countries, our own among them. As to the fact of speaking while in the condition known as trance, or immediately on emerging from it, there appears to be no doubt. Many such have come within my own personal experience in which no claim to spiritualistic influence was put forward. And the "camp meetings," and "protracted meetings," and "love feasts," and "revivals" of our day seldom pass without one or more examples. It must be confessed, however, that the liability to such performances is diminishing every year.

As a manifestation of hysteroid disease, trance-speaking is of decided pathological interest, and will engage our attention hereafter; but the men and women—mostly women—who go about the country talking nonsense and calling it inspired, are the veriest humbugs of the age. I have had the opportunity of hearing these impostors give utterance to language purporting to come from Socrates, Plato, Julius Cæsar, George Washington, Napoleon Bonaparte and other celebrated person-

* Frost's Lives of the Conjurors, London, 1876, p. 199.

ages, in which there were not half a dozen ideas which could be understood, and in which the English tongue, both in its orthography and syntax, was tortured to a degree exceeding the vagaries of Mark Twain and Josh Billings; and yet such men as Mr. Alfred Wallace, who ought to know better, can quote page after page of the stuff uttered by Mrs. Emma Hardinge and extol it to the skies for its miraculous depth and beauty!

Upon one occasion, while a so-called "trance medium" was dilating upon the beauties of the "summer land," in an assumed state of insensibility, I took the liberty of treading on her foot as it rested under the table, and which, as I had seen, exhibited unmistakable evidence of having a large bunion on it. The foot was at once quickly withdrawn, there was unmistakable contortion of the countenance and a very emphatic "Oh!" escaped from the lips. The current of the discourse was interrupted, and when resumed touched upon Hell, or "Hades" as she called it, to which I have no doubt she in her heart consigned all inquiring unbelievers. Now if this woman had been in a condition of trance, my action would have been unfelt, and I would have obtained indubitable evidence of the existence of an abnormal condition of her nervous system and of her sincerity, though of course not of the manifestation being due to spiritual agency.

We have only to look at these people while they are delivering their discourses, to be convinced that they are committing frauds upon their hearers. In actual trance or ecstasy the expression of the face is peculiar and well marked; it is one which no physician who has ever seen a case could fail to recognize, and the attitude and bearing of the subject are such as show unconsciousness. Yet these spiritual trance-mediums stand up before us, acting and looking like other people and tell us they are in a trance and do not know what they are saying! To attempt further to controvert such palpable deception would be almost an insult to the reader's intelligence.

CHAPTER X.

CURING MEDIUMS.

OF all the forms of mediumistic interference, that of healing disease has probably the fullest scope, and for various reasons has most effect with ordinary individuals; and at all times within the historic period there have been persons pretending to supernatural power in curing the ills to which mankind are subject. The fact that success has often followed their performances has given them more or less of the prestige which so generally attends upon the obtainment of favorable results in any direction of effort. It is, however, a very easy matter to dissipate the cloud of mystery which envelops such proceedings, and to show that whatever good fortune has ensued to the subjects who have been operated upon, is due to well-known and very commonplace causes.

The influence by which so-called supernatural cures have been effected has been ascribed to various sources, according to the time at which the healers have performed. At one period it is the direct power of some deity which produces the cure, at another the machinations of devils; again it is the sanctity which resides in the touch of a king, the holiness of a saint, or the superior virtue and godliness of certain other persons; then it is magnetism, and again spiritualism; sometimes it is a peculiar power inherent in some particular person, and at others the direct interference of God for the relief of those who have propitiated him by prayer. Nor does the matter stop here: the bones and other relics of Saints, the halter with which a criminal had been hanged, the moss growing from a dead man's skull, the touch of a dead man's hand, especially of one who had been executed; the heart of a mule ripped up alive, the lungs of a person who had died a violent death, decoctions and powders made from snakes, toads scorpions, etc., and according to St. Augustine an efficacious process employed by the devil was: "*agentis cum patientibus conjungunt, colliger semina serum, eaque materiæ applicam.*"

To trace all these various forms of delusion through their devious courses, though interesting as presenting an important phase of human error, would carry us further than the limits of this work will allow. It will be sufficient for the purpose I have in view to examine into a few of the more prominent, especially as a parity of reasoning can be shown to be applicable to the others.

And to begin with the power of saints and kings to banish disease by a word, a look, or a touch, or even by a visit of the patient to their tombs, or by the efficacy residing in their dead bones, or in the garments they are said to have worn.

According to Görres * the most remarkable instance of curative power possessed by a saint is that afforded by St. Sauveur of Horta. This holy man was born in Catalonia, and received the first part of his name from a presentiment on the part of his sponsors that he was to be a saviour of men, and the second from the fact of his entering a monastery in Horta.

* *Op. Cit.*, t. 1. p 470.

In a fortunate moment the people seemed to have imbibed the idea intuitively that he was possessed of the wonderful gift of healing; for in a short time after he had finished his noviciate, patients came in crowds to Horta from all parts of the country, so that in one single day there were more than two thousand assembled in one place. St. Sauveur was not dismayed; he cured them all, and blessed them in the name of the Holy Trinity, after they had confessed and partaken of Christ's Body. He continued during several years curing those who came to him, and at one time, during the feast of the Annunciation he cured six thousand. But this was not the greatest feat; for another time, at Valencia, in the square before the convent of St. Marie de Jesus, he found more than ten thousand patients, from the viceroy to the laborer, waiting for his benediction and to be cured of their diseases.

Now notwithstanding the great success which St. Sauveur is asserted to have had, he does not seem to have made friends of his brother monks. They became weary of the disorder and dirt caused by so many people coming to the convent. So on one occasion when the bishop came to visit them they complained of their healing brother; and his lordship having no faith—for there were skeptics, then as now, high in ecclesiastical dignity—in St. Sauveur, called the chapter together, summoned him before it, and thus addressed him: "I had hoped to find peace in this house, but on the contrary I meet with trouble, and on your account. Tell me then, brother Sauveur, who has authorized you to live in this manner. Are you not ashamed of hearing people saying 'come let us go to the saint at Horta!' It would be better for them to say 'come to the evil spirit who troubles the brethren at Horta.' But you, my brothers, have done wrong in assuming that he alone could work miracles, for you are just as holy as he. But I will take care, my brother, that your name will not be bandied around in future, for I am going to put an end to your miracles and all these crowds of people. And first, for penance you will receive discipline, then you will change your name to Alphonse, and at midnight you will depart for the monastery of Reus without another word."

Sauveur went to the church without making any reply, and then at the hour that had been fixed upon he set out for the monastery of Reus with a lay brother, passing in silence through the crowd that was collected around the monastery of Horta. He made the journey plunged in fervent prayer.

Arrived at Reus he was received by the abbot with these words: "In order to keep you from disturbing the brothers with your miracles I will put you in a place where you will not be able to incommode them. Go to the kitchen and work your miracles with the plates and dishes."

But the following morning, as soon as it was day, the people of the place came in crowds to the number of more than two thousand, and the sick among them demanded to see brother Sauveur. The brothers, who knew nothing about the matter, went to the abbot, and he, running to the kitchen administered a sharp reprimand to the poor brother, who fell on his knees before him. But in the meantime the crowd besieged the gates and the abbot to appease them was obliged to yield to their wishes on condition that they would all go to the church. Then the saint addressed some simple words to them, blessed them in the name of the Father, the Son, and the

Holy Ghost, and at once returned to his kitchen. The great numbers of crutches, bandages and sticks that were left behind testified to the efficacy of the benediction.

But the abbot at this sight cried out, "Do you see with what filthiness this brother fills the church, making it no better than a stable?"

For some time after this the convent was undisturbed, but as soon as the people knew the way to the saint the processions recommenced. To end them the bishop sent him to Barcelona, then to Saragossa and other places; but after a little while, no matter where he was, it was the same thing. Patients came in crowds and camped out in tents when they could obtain no other shelter.

A still more determined effort was finally made to stop Sauveur's miracles by sending him to Cagliari in Sardinia, but it was the same there as it had been in Spain. Simple, open, in his relations with men, austere towards himself, having no want for a cell, as he passed his nights in prayer in the church, and sleeping, when nature required this indulgence, in a corner of the monastery, Sauveur went on doing his work in the kitchen, the garden, or at the gate distributing alms and blessing the people. He preserved his chastity during all the forty-seven years of his life, though often tempted; his patience and resignation never became less under the many persecutions to which he was subjected; he was compassionate towards the poor and the sick, and full of zeal for the conversion of sinners; he had ecstasies, and frequent visions, especially before the image of the Blessed Virgin, and often while in that state was lifted up in the air in presence of many thousand witnesses. He had the gifts of prophecy, of knowing secret things and of commanding the elements; and in his simplicity was the wonder of his time. The number of patients of all kinds that he cured is incredible. He even resuscitated three dead persons. Finally he died in 1527 (why, is not very evident) after having predicted the exact hour of his death. And even to this day miracles are performed at his tomb.

In view of all that is here said in favor of St. Sauveur, it would be interesting to learn what his brethren and ecclesiastical superiors had to report of his wonderful performances. It is very evident that he was not in favor with them. Certainly if there had been no doubt of the truth of his alleged cures, they would have cherished him, as one able to give great renown to their religious houses, and glory to the Church. And if the history given of him by Görres is only partially true, his memory would have not so entirely gone out of the records of the past as only to be embalmed in a few books on the lives of the Saints. Facts do not disappear so completely. If St. Sauveur had really been the great healer he is said to have been, we should find his doings recorded in a thousand contemporaneous volumes and every schoolboy would have them at his tongue's end. Neither do facts go begging for believers, nor will they remain concealed in obscure books. I have questioned ten educated and intelligent Catholic gentlemen relative to St. Sauveur and not one of them had ever heard of him! How will it be with curing mediums three hundred years hence?

But the mere facts of notoriety and acceptance of assumed miraculous acts are of course no evidence of such acts having been really performed. The belief in the veracity and power of the oracles lasted from far back in the history of Egypt till the time of Theodosius of Greece—several thousand years—and then the temples were closed. Would they have been closed at all if the oracular utterances had really been what was pretended?

Now I have no reason to doubt that many persons were cured by St. Sauveur through their imaginations, and of such diseases as are known can be dispelled by such agency. The bishops and abbots who disciplined him doubtless took this fact into full consideration, and one of the former was certainly right when he said that all the other brethren were just as capable as he of working miracles. But St. Sauveur had somehow got the start and had obtained the power by which such deeds in miraculous therapeutics are done—the confidence of those subjected to treatment—and hence his success.

At the present day we hear very little of cures by ecclesiastical functionaries. Other agencies equally miraculous have taken their place one, by one, and ere long these will also disappear to make room for others doubtless as little founded on truth.

The asserted power of sovereigns, to cure diseases, especially scrofula, by the royal touch, is another example of the rise and fall of a superstitious belief.

The practice appears to have begun with Edward the Confessor, of England, and to have lasted with more or less intensity till the accession of the House of Brunswick, the last sovereign to touch for scrofula having been Anne.

According to other authorities, however, it originated with the early French kings, and there was for a long time a great dispute between writers of England and France relative to the possession of the power—the English denying it to the French kings and the French with equal vigor restricting it to their own sovereigns.

Queen Elizabeth with her hard sense, was very much averse to the practice, though public opinion required her to continue it. Upon one occasion, she told a multitude of the afflicted who besieged her that "God alone could cure their diseases."

During the reign of Charles II. the practice was at its height and yet more deaths took place from scrofula—or king's evil, as it had got to be called—in his reign than in that of any previous sovereign. With Anne the faith which had been held in the efficacy of the royal touch died out, Dr. Samuel Johnson was among the last to receive the imposition of the Queen's hands, which was in his case at least entirely inefficacious, as he was subject to scrofula all his life.

Henry VIII. was the first monarch to establish a particular ceremony to be observed. This was altered at various times, and was printed in the Book of Common Prayer used during the reign of Queen Anne.

With the touch it was customary to give a piece of gold, which was hung around the patient's neck by the sovereign. The desire to get this gold was the cause of many presenting themselves, who were not afflicted with scrofula, and of others repeatedly coming forward. The coins were often found in the shops, having been sold by the recipients. Stringent measures were therefore taken to prevent imposition on the monarch, and after the reign of Elizabeth the size of the coin was reduced.

The form employed by Charles II. is thus described by Evelyn: *

6. [July 1660] "His Majestie first began to *touch for the evil* according to costume, thus—His majestie sitting under his state in the Banquetting House, the Chirurgeons cause the sick to be brought or led up to the throne, where they kneeling, the King strokes their faces or cheekes with both his hands at once, at which instant a Chaplaine in his formalities says: 'He put his hands on them and he healed them:' This is sayed to every one in particular. When they have all been touched they come up againe in the same order; and the other Chaplaine kneeling, and having angel-gold strung on white ribbon on his arme, delivers them one by one to his Majestie, who puts them about the necks of the touched as they passe, whilst the first Chaplaine repeats: 'That is the true light who came into the world.' Then follows an Epistle (as at first, a Gospel) with the Liturgy, prayers for the sick with some alteration, lastly the blessing; and the Lo. Chamberlaine and Comptroller of the Household, bring a basin, ewer and towel for his Majestie to wash."

But there were skeptics, and gradually they outnumbered the believers, and the practice was discontinued on the death of Anne. Among the unbelievers was Mr. Charles Bernard, surgeon, who on being made sergeant-surgeon to the queen became a convert to the doctrine of the efficacy of the royal touch. As Oldmixon † says:

"Yesterday the queen was graciously pleased to touch for the King's evil some particular persons in private; and three

* Memoirs, Chandos Library Edition, London, p. 266.

† History of England, Vol. II. p. 302.

weeks after, December 19, yesterday, about twelve at noon her Majesty was pleased to touch, at St. James', about twenty persons afflicted with the King's evil. The more ludicrous sort of skeptics, in this case, asked why it was not called the queen's evil, as the chief court of justice was called the Queen's Bench. But Charles Bernard, the surgeon who had made this touching the subject of his raillery all his lifetime till he became body surgeon at court, and found it a good perquisite, solved all difficulties by telling his companions with a fleer '*Really one could not have thought it, if one had not seen it.*' A friend of mine heard him say it, and knew well his opinion of it."

As we have seen, the French kings also touched for scrofula, and it is claimed by some, that the practice originated with them. Servetus, who was not of a credulous mind, says in the first edition of his "Ptolemy" published in 1535, that he had seen the king touch many persons for the disease, but he had never seen any that were cured thereby.* But the last clause of this sentence excited the ire of the censor, and in the next edition published in 1541, the words "*an sanati fuerint non vidi*" were changed to "*pluresque sanatos passim audivi.*" I have heard of many that were cured. Testimony in support of miracles has often been manufactured, but the natural obstinacy and truthfulness of Servetus would not admit of his giving his personal endorsement at the expense of his convictions.

It is very certain that if there had been any real efficacy as such in the royal touch the practice would never have been discontinued. That cases were cured by it is probable, just as

* "Vidi ipse Regem plurimos hoc languore correptos tangentem, an sanati fuerint non vidi."

they are cured by any imposing ceremony, or action, or thing that appeals to the imagination and rouses the spirit of hope. But the respect for kings and queens which once existed in an extreme degree, began to fade out after its spasmodic revival with the restoration of the monarchy in England, and hence, reaching its acme with Charles II., touching gradually lost its hold on the people, along with many other notions pertaining to the "divine right of kings." But it held its sway for over seven hundred years—to be utterly extinguished at last—a type doubtless of many other delusions which still prevail to a greater or less extent.

The relics of saints and holy men and women of all religions have in former times enjoyed a very high reputation for their sanitary virtues. At the present day they are at a discount with all civilized nations, except among the ignorant and superstitious, and whole communities reject all idea of their efficacy, substituting, however, very often, some other equally absurd belief.

The therapeutical influence supposed to be attached to the tombs of such persons, like that associated with relics, is not so powerful as it once was. Credulity runs in other channels, and for the same reason we do not now use dead men's skulls, or their dried livers, or mummified reptiles in our therapeutics.

But supernatural powers of healing were claimed by others in virtue of some special gift with which they and their followers asserted them to be endowed. Among these was Mr. Valen tine Greatrix or Greatreakes, who obtained great celebrity during the reign of Charles II., as a curer, by the touch, of ague, epilepsy, paralysis, deafness, and other affections of the nervous system more or less under the influence of the emotions and of the imagination.

Another was Prince Hohenlohe, who likewise operated on convulsions, paralysis, deafness, blindness, etc., and who even still is regarded by some persons as a veritable worker of miracles.

Again, there was George Fox, the founder of the Quakers, whose single case, though very striking at the time, was like the greater part of those relieved by similar means, only temporary in its duration. He thus records it.*

" After some time I went to the meeting at Arnside where Richard Meyer was. Now he had been long lame of one of his arms; and I was moved by the Lord to say unto him, among all the people, ' Prophet Meyer stand up upon thy legs, (for he was sitting down) and he stood up and stretched out his arm that had been lame a long time, and said: ' Be it known unto all you people that this day I am healed.' But his parents could hardly believe it, but after the meeting was done, had him aside and took off his doublet; and then they saw it was true. He soon after came to Swarthmore meeting, and there declared how that the Lord had healed him. But after this the Lord commanded him to go to York with a message from him; and he disobeyed the Lord; and the Lord struck him again, so that he died about three-quarters of a year after."

There are many other persons who might be mentioned in illustration, but their examples would teach us nothing new relative to the matter in question.

* Journal, Vol. I. p. 103, London, 1794. Cited by Pettigrew in "Superstitions connected with the History and Practice of Medicine." London 1844, p. 116.

Mesmerism or animal magnetism has put forward strong claims to be regarded as a curative agent, and if we look at the subject from a proper stand-point we will find reasons, as in all the other alleged instances, to admit certain facts as being sufficiently well established. But experience and careful investigation show that all such cures are to be ascribed to emotional disturbance, to imagination, to hypnotism or artificial sleep, to expectant attention, to suggestion or some other well-known principle. Some thirty years ago a mesmeric infirmary was established in London, and many cases of disease were treated there; and by mesmeric operators, in other parts of England, cases were reported as being cured. The affections, however, were of the nervous system, or were self-limited, or were of such a character as to allow of errors in diagnosis on the part of the ignorant persons, many of them laymen, who undertook the cures.

For instance, I have before me a number of the "*Zoist, a Journal of Cerebral Physiology and Mesmerism, and their applications to Human Welfare,*"* edited by Dr. Elliotson, a learned but credulous physician, who for a time, fought with great vigor in support of the doctrines he had embraced Though at first mesmerism gained many adherents from Dr. Elliotson's association with it, even his name was not sufficient. Its followers deserted in large numbers, the infirmary was closed, and Dr. Elliotson himself sank into comparative obscurity.

But to return to the "Zoist."

The cases of cure reported in the number referred to—and

* October, 1851.

it is a fair sample of all the others—are "Good Effect of Mesmerism in an Epileptic Fit." "Striking Proofs of the remedial Power of Mesmerism over Epilepsy," "Cure of a Case of Insanity," "Cure of a most intense Nervous Affection commonly called Spinal Irritation," "Cures of Loss of Voice, Neuralgia, Spinal Irritation, Excruciating Rheumatism," "Cure of a large Polypus of the Uterus."

And this is a sample of the cures. It is reported by a Mr. Masset, Jr.

"I was walking out on Thursday evening the 13th when I saw a crowd; and upon asking what was the matter was informed that there was a woman dying who had been taken into the stable adjoining the inn called the "Baldfaced Stag." I went in and found a woman in fits, foaming at the mouth. A policeman of Highgate had hold of her by one arm, and two laborers held the other. She was struggling against them with all her might. I immediately without asking questions, commenced making passes downwards from her head to her feet, and in *less than two minutes* she was quite calm. I made the men leave hold of her, and then she complained of pains in her side. These I relieved *instantly* by local passes on the place she pointed out to me. I then instantly threw her into a beautiful, calm sleep, and she remained quite still; her breathing being hardly visible. I left her, and calling on the following morning found her *in the same attitude in which I had left her.* The men who had slept on some straw by her side all night (one of them was her husband) told me that she had walked thirty miles, and that she often had fits, but that she had slept well all night. I ordered some breakfast for her and left her, and have not heard of them since."

Every physician will at once see all the fallacious points of this case; but others who may read this work may run some risk of being deceived with an account which to a person unacquainted with the phenomenon of epilepsy appears to relate a cure of this terrible disease. I will therefore say:

1st. That the convulsive stage of an epileptic paroxysm, if left to itself, rarely lasts over two or three minutes. This was one of the exceptions, as it continued much longer—two minutes in fact after Mr. Masset began his passes.

2d. That stupor almost invariably follows severe epileptic convulsions and often lasts several hours. Besides she had walked thirty miles and was consequently tired and disposed to sleep.

3d. The woman had had repeated attacks before, from which she recovered without treatment.

4th. Physicians who understand their profession employ no treatment for the simple uncomplicated epileptic paroxysm, knowing that the natural tendency is for it to cease spontaneously. I have seen hundreds of cases in which just such phenomena existed as in Mr. Masset's case, and in which there was no treatment beyond putting something between the teeth to prevent injury to the tongue and cheeks.

5th. The cure of epilepsy consists not in arresting a paroxysm which has already begun, but in preventing the occurrence of others.

It is however with perfect truth that Dr. Elliotson states in a note that had Mr. Masset done this in former days he would in due time have been canonized. It was just such cures as his that led to the canonization of their performers, and just such, produced by mesmerizers and spiritualists of the present day, that excite the astonishment of the credulous and ignorant.

Dr. Ashburner's "Cure of a large Polypus of the Uterus" was effected by his mesmerizing the patient for at least an hour every day and pointing the fingers of his right hand at her eyes for half an hour daily. In eight weeks the tumor was gone. The patient had suffered from profuse hemorrhage from the uterus; and the symptoms were indicative of a miscarriage rather than a polypus. But even if there were a polypus, spontaneous cure after profuse hemorrhage is a well known occasional circumstance. Dr. Ashburner's cure of it by pointing his fingers at the patient's eyes is about on a par with a person standing by a railroad track pointing his hand at a passing train, and then reporting that he had by that action caused the movement of the engine.

But the mesmerizers do not limit their therapeutical operations to the human species. Mr. H. S. Thomson * contributes to the "*Zoist*" an account of cures of two horses, one of a sore eye and the other of an inflamed leg, by passes made over the diseased parts.

A still more remarkable case in the eyes of the faithful is that which occurred in Miss Martineau's experience, and which I quote in the language of the estimable reporter.†

"BOLTON NEAR SKIPTON,
"August 19, 1850.

"DEAR DR. ELLIOTSON,

"Your note has just reached me having been forwarded from home. The story of the cow is this. One very hot even-

* No xii., p. 522.

† "*Zoist*," Oct. 1850, No. xxxi., p. 301.

ing in July I took some young cousins to see my stock, and I saw a small pail half full of blood at the door of the cow's house. During my absence that day my cow Ailsie had been taken violently ill, so that the servants had sent to Rydal for the cow-doctor, who had bled her and given her strong medicines. This had been done some hours before I saw her, and the doctor said that if she was not much relieved before his evening visit, he was sure she would die. There were no signs of relief in any way when I saw her at seven o'clock, nor when the doctor came soon after eight. He said she could not recover and it was a chance if she lived till morning. At ten she was worse, and to be sure no creature could appear in a more desperate state. She was struggling for breath, quivering, choking and all in a flame of fire. Her eyes were starting; her mouth and nostrils dry; and the functions suspended, as they had been all day.

"It occurred to me then, to have her mesmerized; but I am afraid I was rather ashamed. The man knew nothing whatever about mesmerism except the fact that I had once done it with success to his sister. I believe he had not the remotest idea what was done or what it meant.

"I desired him to come up to the house at twelve o'clock and let me know Ailsie's state. As I sat during these two hours I remembered how I had known cats affected by mesmerism, and how Sullivan the whisperer tamed vicious horses, and Catlin learned from the Indians how to secure buffalo calves by what seemed clearly to be mesmerism, and I determined to try it upon the cow if by midnight she proved to be past the power of medicine.

"At midnight I went down and found that there was no

improvement or promise of any. I then directed the man to mesmerize her, and showed him how. He was to persevere till he saw some change, in making passes along the spine from the head to the tail, and also across the chest, as she labored more dreadfully than ever in her breathing. Within a few minutes her breathing became easier, her eyes less wild, her mouth moist, and before morning she was relieved in all ways.

"The first news I heard was of the astonishment of the Rydal doctor, who came early without an idea that she could be alive. He exclaimed that he had 'never thought to see her alive again,' that 'it was a good £10 in Miss M.'s pocket,' and so forth. One thing struck me much. My man called to me when I was in the garden and asked me to come and see how 'Ailsie fare to go to sleep like' when he mesmerized her, and it really was curious to see how her eyes grew languid and gradually closed under the treatment.

"This was not all. Towards noon I was told that Ailsie had relapsed and was almost as bad as ever. I went down and saw that it was so, and ordered an hour's mesmerizing again. The relief was as striking as before, and in two hours more she was out of danger, and has been very well since.

"I foresee how such a story may be ridiculed; but I perceive how important it is that we should gather some facts about the power of mesmerizing our brutes; not only for truth's and humanity's sake, but because the establishment of a few such facts would dispose of the objection that the results of mesmerism are all imagination. I am fond of my cow and stand up for her good qualities, but I cannot boast of any imaginative faculty in her. A cow morbidly imaginative is a new idea I believe. If it is true that the greatest chemist in the world says that he must believe if he saw a baby mesmerized, I would ask him whether a cow, or a cat, or a vicious horse would not do as well."

"If my cows are ever ill again I will try the experiment with great care and let you know the result. I may mention that some of my neighbors were aware of the desperate illness of the cow; and of her doctor's astonishment at her recovery. We did not tell the doctor how we interfered with his patient, and I dare say he has not heard of it at this hour, but others of my neighbors were deeply interested in the story and wished it could be made known. To this I can have no objection, as I do not mind a laugh, and should be glad to save the life of even a single cow.

"I am, dear Dr. Elliotson, yours truly,

"HARRIET MARTINEAU."

That animals as well as men can be put into the condition of hypnotism or artificial somnambulism is well known, and will be fully considered in a subsequent part of this book. But if the curative influence of mesmerism were as strong as Miss Martineau and Dr. Elliotson supposed, we should not now see the practice confined to the merest ignoramuses and charlatans which the world is capable of producing. Miss Martineau's recital simply presents another example of a fact "viewed unequally." One of those in which all the conditions which might have acted in curing the cow independently of mesmerism, are not eliminated. Thus the animal may have been cured by the cow-doctor, or may have spontaneously recovered, the disease—probably pneumonia—having run its course. Certainly if mesmerism were capable of exercising such immediate and striking influence as Miss Martineau supposes, it would not now be disregarded as a healing agent. There is no difficulty in getting physicians to accept all means of curing their patients which experience show to be useful; but knowing the falsity of the claims put forward in behalf of nine out of ten of the agents whose therapeutical power is vaunted, they naturally fight shy of such things at first.

It is very certain that all the truth of mesmerism as a healing agent is accepted by the medical profession. Thus the ability to produce artificial somnambulism in some patients is not questioned, nor the fact that during its existence surgical operations can be performed without causing pain to the subject. These are matters that admit of demonstration, and they have been demonstrated. But the mind of a well trained and thoroughly educated physician accepts nothing as fact till it is proven, and it is the persistent and unreasonable attempts of the adherents of theories, to command his acceptance of their doctrines on insufficient evidence, and often on no evidence at all, that excites his spirit of opposition and contempt. He does not cease to remember that proof and assertion are two very different things.

Dr. Elliotson * when he cites the following story does so as an instance of an impossibility; but I think I will be able to show that it relates to an event which is no more impossible than Miss Martineau's cure of the cow.

Voltaire advises the devil never to address himself to the faculty of physic, but to that of theology, when he wishes to impose upon mankind. However, in 1726 a poor woman at

* Human Physiology Fifth edition, London, p. 672. Also "*Zoist*," October, 1851, p. 235.

Godalming in Surrey, pretended that after a violent longing for rabbits while pregnant, she brought forth these animals; and persuaded her apothecary, Mr. Howard, a man of probity who had practised for thirty years, or in common language, a highly respectable practitioner of great experience, that in the course of about a month he had delivered her of about twenty rabbits. George the First, not thinking it impossible, sent his house surgeon, Mr. Akers, to inquire into the fact, and the royal house surgeon returned to London convinced that he had obtained *ocular* and *tangible* proof of the truth, and promised to procure the woman a pension. The wise king then sent his sergeant-surgeon, Mr. St. André, and the sergeant-surgeon returned to town a firm believer. They both returned with rabbits as proof, and the rabbits had the high honor of being dissected before the king. An elaborate report of the production and dissection was published by the sergeant-surgeon, and the honest, severe, vain and visionary Arian clergyman Whiston, (of the faculty of theology indeed) in a pamphlet (for a furious controversy arose between the believers and the unbelievers), *showed* that it was an exact fulfilment of a prophecy in Esdras. An eminent physician, Sir Richard Manningham, backed by Caroline, the Princess of Wales, detected the cheat, and on the threat of a dangerous operation and imprisonment, Mary Tofts confessed the fraud.

These are Dr. Elliotson's own words, italics and all, and he cites the case as an actual impossibility. But there are no impossibilities outside the domain of pure mathematics, and I contend that not only is Mary Tofts' case not an impossibility, but that it is fully as probable as most of the more astonishing manifesta tions of mesmerism, spiritualism, or any other pseudo science.

1. In the first place it is not unique. Bartholinus * states that Johannes Naboronsky, a noble Pole and his good friend, told him at Basel, that he had seen in Poland, two fish without scales, which were born from a woman, and that as soon as they were delivered they were put into water, where they swam about like other fish.

The same veracious and honest chronicler gives his testimony to the fact that a woman of good quality at Elsinghorn, being about to be confined, prepared everything for the event. In due time labor ensued, and after much travail she gave birth to a creature resembling a large dormouse; which, to the great amazement of the women who were present, with wonderful agility sought and found a hole in the chamber, into which it entered, and was never seen afterwards.

And again; that in the year 1639, in Norway, occurred the remarkable case of a woman, who, the mother of several children, again being in labor, was delivered of two eggs, like hens' eggs in every respect. One of these eggs was broken, but the other was sent to the famous Dr. Olaus Wormius, who kept it in his museum, where all who wished might see it. In support of this history he adduces the following certificate.

"We, whose names are hereunto written, Ericus Westergard, Rotolph Rakertad and Thor Venes, coadjutors of the pastor in the parish of Niæss, do certify to all men, that anno 1639, upon the twentieth day of May (by command of the Lord President in Remerige, the Lord Paulus Tranius, pastor in Niæss) we went to receive an account of the monstrous birth in Sundby; brought forth by an honest woman, Anna, the

* Anatomicæ institutiones corporis humani utriusque sexus historiam, etc. Lugduni Batavorum hist. 66, p. 103.

daughter of Amundus the wife of Gudbandus Erlandsonius, who already had been the mother of eleven children, the last of which she was delivered of upon the fourth of March, 1638. This Anna in the year 1639, upon the seventh of April began to grow ill; and being in great pain in her belly, she caused her neighbors to be called in to her assistance; the same day, about the evening, in the presence of her neighbors, she brought forth an egg, in all respects like that of a hen, which being broken by the women present, Anna Grimen, Ellen Rudstad, Gyro Rudstad and Catharina Sunby, they found that in it the yolk and white answered directly to a common egg. Upon the eighteenth day of April, about noon, in the presence of the same people, she was delivered of another egg, which in figure was nothing different from the former. The mother reported this to us; the women that assisted at her delivery confirmed the truth of it; as also that the pains of this birth had been more sharp to her than all the rest of the former. That this was the confession, as well of the mother as of them that were present, we do attest with our seals in the presence of the Lord President, in the parish of Niæss, the day and year abovesaid."*

The great Wormius looked upon this as a diabolical work, since by the artifice of the devil many other things are conveyed into and formed in the bodies of men and women.

Here we have the testimony of eye witnesses, of a commission of clergymen, of Wormius, one of the most distinguished of anatomists, besides that of the woman herself and the actual existence of the egg in the museum of a University Can mesmerism and spiritualism do better?

* "Wonders of the Little World," by Nathaniel Wanley, London, 1806.

And further in support of the alleged fact that women are at times, like birds and most reptiles, oviparous, we have testimony to the effect that the women of the Selenetidæ, unlike other women, lay eggs from which men are hatched, and the learned Lycosthenes,* in referring to the circumstance which he accepts as a fact, gives an illustration which, as going into details, and therefore adding to the testimony, I subjoin.

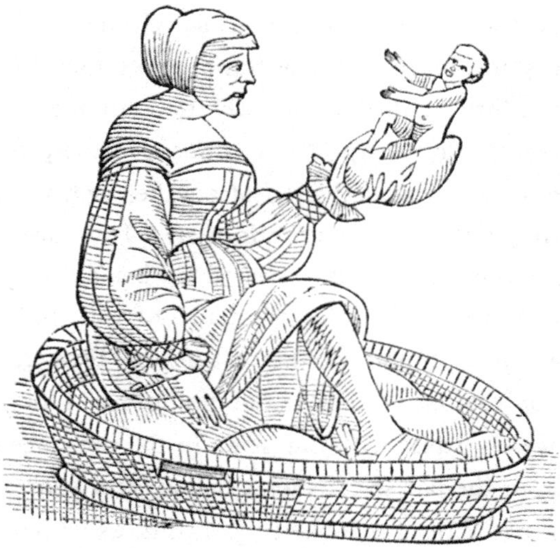

Fig. 5.

Franciscus Rossetus † says:

"Anne Tromperin, the wife of a certain porter in our hospital, being about thirty years of age, was delivered of a boy and two serpents upon St. John's day, anno 1576. She told me upon her faith 'That in the summer before, in an

* Prodigiorum ac ostentorum chronicon, etc, Basileæ, 1557, p. 13.

† De Partu Cæsareo, Basileæ, 1582. Waniey, p. 282.

extreme hot day, she had drank of a spring if the grove called Brudetholk, a place within a quarter of a mile from Basel, where she suspected she had drank of the sperm of serpents.' She afterwards grew so big that she was fain to carry her belly in a swathing band. The child was so lean that he was scarcely anything but bones. The serpents were each of them an ell long and as thick as the arm of an infant, both of which, alive as they were, were buried by the midwife in the church-yard of St. Elizabeth."

Many other examples to the like effect might readily be adduced, but the foregoing are sufficient to establish the precedent of women giving birth to the lower animals; and hence to show that the case which Dr. Elliotson considers an impossibility, is supported by analogous instances.

2. In the second place we have to inquire into the character of the evidence offered in support of the alleged births of rabbits by Mary Tofts.

Three medical gentlemen of the highest respectability, visited and examined the woman and obtained some of the rabbits. The king himself saw them, and they were dissected and shown to be veritable rabbits. Besides this, a distinguished clergyman demonstrated from scripture the fact that the event did take place, and that it was in fulfilment of a prophecy. When science and theology agree, surely the probability of error is rendered exceedingly small.

3. The confession of Mary Tofts to the effect that she had committed a fraud, is the strongest point yet adduced tending to show that she did not commit a fraud.

The confession was made under threats of a painful operation and punishment. Every jurist knows of how little value a confession is, when extorted by such means. Mary Tofts would doubtless under like compulsion have acknowledged herself to be a witch or anything else that her questioners might have desired. "As if" to quote Beccaria,* "truth resided in the muscles and fibres of a wretch in torture."

Besides, confessions are made continually, every time a flagrant crime is committed, by persons seeking notoriety, or some other end, or from delusion, or other morbid impulse. What more likely, than that Mary Tofts was driven into insanity by the questionings to which she was subjected, and by the agitation into which she was thrown at the idea of the contest which was urged relative to the reality of her lepurine delivery?

I think therefore it will be admitted that the evidence in favor of Mary Tofts is much stronger than that adduced in support of Miss Martineau; and yet Dr. Elliotson declares the one to have been guilty of fraud, while the other is held up as a pattern of nobility and goodness!

Spiritualism has not been especially distinguished for its remarkable cures, although it puts forward pretensions to powerful therapeutical influence. Occasionally we hear of some travelling charlatan who pretends to the possession of specific healing virtue, and who by impressing the imaginations of his ignorant *clientelle*, or by telling them in a loud and imperious voice, that they are cured, or by knocking them down and then bidding them rise and find their maladies gone, succeeds, sometimes, in relieving patients of certain affections of the nervous system; or of persuading them for a time that

* "An Essay on Crimes and Punishment." Translated from the Italian, with the Commentary of Voltaire. London 1801, p. 56.

they were relieved. Many of these latter have come under my notice with their diseases unmitigated, and in whom the belief of a cure had been effected solely by the principle of suggestion, which the electro-biologist knows so well how to use.

Again, many of the sick who resort to clairvoyant and spiritualistic humbugs, have their maladies temporarily relieved through the emotional disturbance consequent on visiting such people, who always preserve a certain air of mystery well calculated to impress the ignorant. In such cases the abatement of the symptoms, has its analogue in the fact that a mere visit to the dentist often cures a raging tooth-ache. The clairvoyant or spiritualistic quack takes advantage of the period of momentary relief which the patient experiences, and of the gratitude which all patients temporarily feel when freed from suffering, to get a certificate setting forth the fact; and this is speedily published as a bait for other credulous sufferers.

The influence of the imagination in curing disease has already engaged a good portion of our attention, but the subject is very extensive, and can scarcely be touched in any of its relations without leading to interesting illustrations.

Thus about seventy or eighty years ago, an American named Perkins excited great interest in this country, and in England and France, by curing diseases by the use of little metallic rods, which he called tractors, from the fact that they were drawn over the diseased part. Many were apparently healed by them, but they fell into disrepute as soon as Dr. Haygarth demonstrated from numerous examples, that wooden tractors, painted to look like the metallic ones, were fully as efficacious.

Then, quite recently, was the metal-cure of Dr. Burq * of Paris, which was endorsed by Dr. Elliotson, who was capable of believing everything but that women could conceive rabbits. As another instance of human folly, I give the following account of this delusion, which, I think, has never taken root in this country.

In 1847, Dr. Burq, as he says, noticed in a woman whom he was mesmerizing for hysteria and phthisis, in the hospital Beaujon, that as often as she was thrown into a mesmeric sleep, the direct contact of certain metals was insupportable. while that of others was agreeable to the touch, or at least, caused no signs of repugnance. If, for instance, he suddenly placed a piece of copper, iron or steel on her bare hand, or any other part of her body, she instantly, and sometimes in the midst of the apparently deepest sleep, repelled it roughly, often with an expression of suffering, or even of anger if the experiment was repeated too frequently. If a key, or a shovel, or iron tongs were placed upon her bed near enough to her to make their influence felt, she instantly discovered them and got rid of them, either by a sudden movement, if the object were not fixed or large, or with her hand, covered previously with something to insulate it, when a greater or more direct effort was required. The latter precaution was always carefully taken, when, in order to open a door in her sleep-walking, she was under the necessity of slowly turning the key or the handle of the lock.

If, however, gold or silver were placed in her hands, she

* "Nervous Affections. Metallo-therapia, or metal-cure; New properties of metals illustrated through mesmerism." Translated, communicated and supplied with a note, by Dr. Elliotson; "*Zoist*," July and October, 1852.

showed much pleasure in handling them, provided the gold, and especially the silver, was not much alloyed with copper. If it were, her repugnance was in direct ratio to the extent of the debasement of the precious metal.

Dr. Burq was very much astonished at these results; though the exhibition of pleasure in handling gold or silver is no very unusual phenomenon. He determined, therefore, to investigate farther, and accordingly performed the following experiment.

The patient being mesmerized, and her insensibility perfectly proved by a pin being stuck into her skin, he repeatedly applied, to different parts of her body, different pieces of money of nearly equal size. With the copper coins, a few seconds were sufficient to restore sensibility; first in the parts touched by the metal, and then in the surrounding parts; whereas with the gold and silver, nothing of the kind was observed, except when instead of the silver coin, he substituted another piece of the same metal of inferior value by being an alloy.

The patient died a few days afterwards, before Dr. Burq could draw any decided conclusion, but he resolved in spite of many difficulties to pursue the investigation further, and in the course of three years built up the system of practice which he called metal-cure. He asserted that cases of anæsthesia, cramps, paralysis, etc., were cured by different metals, especially if the patient were hysterical. Epilepsy he could not manage at all. Brass was found a very efficacious metal in the treatment of hysteria; the mental quality which goes by that name is also valuable to the practitioner in like cases, and Dr. Burq appears to have had a good stock of both. As Dr.

Elliotson remarks: Dr. Burq, in his memoir entitled "*Mesmerism Illustrated by the Metals*," shows a "remarkable relation which he has discovered between the effects of brass and those of mesmerism."

But notwithstanding the publication of remarkable results, the metal-cure made little headway, and is now almost forgotten; and yet its efficacy was attested by as good evidence as any adduced in favor of mesmerism or spiritualism.

Another delusion, which over two hundred years ago was in high favor, was that relative to the cure of wounds by the "powder of sympathy," as described and advocated by Sir Kenelm Digby.*

The first published case of the effects of this mode of treatment attracted great attention; and as a further contribution, I quote it in Sir Kenelm Digby's own words as he related it in his discourse before the noble and learned assembly he addressed.

"Mr. James Howel (well known in France for his public works, and particularly for his *Dendrologia*, translated into French by Monsieur Baudoin) coming by chance as two of his best friends were fighting a duel, he did his endeavor to part them; and putting himself between them, seized with his left hand upon the hilt of the sword of one of the combatants, while with his right hand he lay hold of the blade of the other; they being transported with fury, one against the other, struggled to rid themselves of the hindrance their friend

* "A late discovery made in a solemne assembly of nobles and learned men, at Montpellier, in France, touching the cure of wounds, by the Powder of Sympathy; with instructions how to make the said Powder, etc." London, 1658.

made that they should not kill one another; and one of them roughly drawing the blade of his sword, cut to the very bone the nerves and muscles of Mr. Howel's hand; and then the other disengaging his hilt, gave a cross blow on his adversary's head, which glanced towards his friend, who heaving up his sore hand to save the blow, he was wounded on the back of his hand as he had been before within. It seems some strange constellation reigned them against him that he should lose so much blood by parting two such dear friends, who, had they been themselves, would have hazarded both their lives to have preserved his; but this involuntary effusion of blood by them, prevented that which they should have drawn one from the other. For they seeing Mr. Howel's face besmeared with blood by heaving up his wounded hand, they both ran to embrace him; and having searched his hurts, they bound up his hand with one of his garters to close the veins which were cut and bled abundantly. They brought him home and sent for a surgeon. But this being heard at court, the king sent one of his own surgeons, for his majesty much affected the said Mr. Howel.

"It was my chance to be lodged hard by him, and four or five days after, as I was making myself ready, he came to my house and prayed me to view his wounds, 'for I understand,' said he, 'that you have extraordinary remedies upon such occasions, and my surgeons apprehend for fear that it may grow to gangrene, and so the hand must be cut off.' In effect his countenance discovered that he was in much pain, which he said was unsupportable in regard of the extreme inflammation; I told him that I would willingly cure him, but if haply he knew the manner how I would cure him, without touching or seeing him, it may be he would not expose himself to my manner of curing, because he would think it, peradventure, either ineffectual or superstitious; he replied that the wonderful things which many have related unto me of your way of curing, makes me nothing doubt at all of its efficacy; and all that I have to say unto you is comprehended in the Spanish proverb '*Hagase el milagro y hagalo Mahoma.*' Let the miracle be done, though Mahomet do it."

"I asked him then for anything that had the blood upon it so he presently sent for his garter wherewith his hand was first bound; and having called for a basin of water, as if I would wash my hands, I took a handful of powder of vitriol which I had in my study, and presently dissolved it. As soon as the bloody garter was brought me, I put it within the basin, observing in the interim what Mr. Howel did, who stood talking with a gentleman in a corner of my chamber, not regarding at all what I was doing; but he started suddenly as if he had found some strange alteration in himself; I asked him what he ailed? I know not what ails me, but I find that I feel no more pain; methinks that a pleasing kind of freshness, as it were a wet cold napkin did spread over my hand, which hath taken away the inflammation that tormented me before. I replied, since that you feel already so good an effect of my medicament, I advise you to cast away all your plasters, only keep the wound clean and in a moderate temper, 'twixt heat and cold. This was presently reported to the Duke of Buckingham, and a little after, to the king, who were both very curious to know the circumstance of the business, which was that after dinner I took the garter out of the water and put it to dry before a great fire. It was scarce dry but Mr.

Howel's servant came running that his master felt as much burning as ever he had done, if not more, for the heat was such as if his hand were 'twixt coals of fire; I answered that although that had happened at present, yet he should find ease in a short time, for I knew the reason of this new accident, and I would provide accordingly, for his master should be free from that inflammation, it may be, before he could possibly return unto him; but in case he found no ease I wished him to come presently back again, if not, he might forbear coming Thereupon he went, and at the instant, I did put again the garter into the water; thereupon he found his master without any pain at all. To be brief, there was no sense of pain afterward, but within five or six days the wounds were cicatrized and entirely healed. King James required a punctual information of what had passed touching this cure; and after it was done and perfected, his majesty would needs know of me how it was done, having drolled with me first (which he could do with a very good grace) about a magician and a sorcerer; I answered that I should be always ready to perform what his majesty should command, but I most humbly desired him, before I should pass further, to tell him what the author of whom I had the secret said to the great Duke of Tuscany upon the like occasion. It was a religious Carmelite that came from the Indies and Persia to Florence, he had also been at China, who having done many marvellous cures with his powder after his arrival to Tuscany, the Duke said he would be very glad to learn it of him. It was the father of the great Duke who governs now. The Carmelite answered him that it was a secret which he had learnt in the oriental parts, and he thought there was not any who knew it in

Europe but himself; and that it deserved not to be divulged, which could not be done if his highness would meddle with it, because he was not likely to do it with his own hands, but must trust a surgeon or some other servant, so that in a short time divers others would côme to know it as well as himself. But a few months after I had an opportunity to do an important courtesy to the said friar, which induced him to discover unto me his secret, and the same year he returned to Persia; insomuch that there is no other knows this secret in Europe but myself. The king replied that he needed not apprehend any fear that he would discover, for he would not trust anybody in the world to make experience of his secret, but he would do it with his own hands; therefore he would have some of the powder; which I delivered, instructing him in all the circumstances. Whereupon his majesty made sundry proofs whence he derived singular satisfaction."

But the king's physician, Dr. Mayerne, watched the royal practitioner and discovered that vitriol was used. Whereupon Sir Kenelm instructed him fully. Dr. Mayerne soon after went to France on a visit to his friend, the Duke of Mayerne, and told him the secret, and thence it soon became generally known, so that Sir Kenelm said it came by degrees "to be so divulged that now there is scarce any country barber but knows it."

Now, as learning was in those days, Sir Kenelm Digby was a learned man, and the object of his discourse was to show, not only that wounds could be healed by his manner of proceeding, but to explain the *rationale* of the process. For this latter purpose he adduced arguments based on the physical properties of light, air, etc., and in the course of his reasoning, brought forward certain alleged phenomena which he thought were analogous in character. It is a very curious circumstance that of these, there is not one which is true. Thus he is wrong when he says that if the hand be severely burnt, the pain and inflammation are relieved by holding it near a hot fire; that a person who has a bad breath, is cured by putting his head over a privy and inhaling the air which comes from it; that those who are bitten by vipers or scorpions, are cured by holding the bruised head of either of those animals, as the case may be, near the bitten part; that in times of great contagion, carrying a toad, or a spider, or arsenic "or some other venomous substance" about the person, is a protection; that hanging a toad about the neck of a horse affected with farcy, dissipates the disease; that water evaporated in a close room will not be deposited on the walls, if a vessel of water be placed in the room; that venison pies smell strongly at those periods in which "the beasts which are of the same nature and kind are in rut;" that wine in the cellar undergoes a fermentation when the vines in the fields are in flower; that a tablecloth spotted with mulberries or red wine is more easily whitened at the season in which the plants are flowering than at any other; that washing the hands in the rays of moonlight which fall into a polished silver basin (without water) is a cure for warts, that a vessel of water put on the hearth of a smoky chimney, is a remedy for the evil, and so on,—not a single fact in all that he adduces. Yet these circumstances were regarded as real, and were spoken of at the time as irrefragable proofs of the truth of Sir Kenelm's views.

Sympathetic cures have long since gone the way of kindred follies, the way which mesmerism has already begun to take, and on which spiritualism will surely enter ere many years have lapsed.

And yet, absurd as it was, we owe to Sir Kenelm Digby's practice one of the greatest improvements in surgery which the world has known. Artificial somnambulism or hypnotism will survive mesmerism; something beneficial may come out of spiritualism; but the curing of wounds by the use of sympathetic powders led to the modern system of healing by the first intention, and thus revolutionized the whole art of surgery, to the inestimable good of the human species.

We have only to refer to the surgical treatises written before Sir Kenelm began to treat wounds, to learn how barbarous, and with our light, how senseless, was the system used before his day. The object was to keep a wound open so that it might discharge itself of its "bad humors," the flow of blood was stopped by pouring into it melted tar or boiling oil, and when operations were performed red hot knives were used so as to prevent hæmorrhage.

But in Sir Kenelm Digby's process the wound was cleaned, the edges were brought together, and it was kept quiet and protected from the atmosphere. By this treatment the cure was greatly facilitated, and as it was attended without the pain accompanying the ordinary process, it grew into favor; and though the treatment by sympathetical powders fell into disrepute, it became the first object of the surgeon to procure union without suppuration.

It has often happened that permanent advances in medical science have resulted from experiments made with quite a different object in view. Thus the discovery of modern anæsthesia by the inhalation of certain vapors, was the direct result of breathing nitrous oxide gas and the vapor of ether for purposes of exhilaration. And local anæsthesia from the application of the ether spray, which was at first supposed to be due to some specific property of the ether, is now known to be caused by the intense cold which ensues. In the other sciences also, great discoveries have been made by the misdirected efforts of eager inquirers. The search for the philosopher's stone constitutes almost the foundation of modern chemistry.

But to return to the cures by spiritualists. In all alleged cases, where the cure is real, imagination or emotional excitement has been the healing agent. Whether the operator be the Zouave Jacob, or Judge Edwards, or Mrs. Emma Hardinge, or "Prof." Brittain, or Andrew Jackson Davis, or Dr. Robert Newton, the influence is the same and resides not in the operator—except in so far as he is able to obtain the confidence of the subject—but in the patient, just as it does in cases of mesmeric, sympathetic, astrological, and other delusional agencies, through the apparent action of which maladies have been cured.

That such cures are unjustifiable I am not prepared to say. The patient, like Mr. Howel to Sir Kenelm Digby, is always ready to exclaim "Let the miracle be done, though Mahomet do it!" Physicians requently banish real or imaginary affections by the use of bread pills, and many a person has been cured by the application of some instrument, as the stethoscope or thermometer, intended only as a means of examination.

Thus Dr. Paris * says that "as soon as the powers of nitrous oxide gas were discovered, Dr. Beddoes at once con-

* Pharmacologia, p. 28.

cluded that it must necessarily be a specific for paralysis; a patient was selected for trial, and the management of it was intrusted to Sir Humphrey Davy. Previous to the administration of the gas, he inserted a small thermometer under the tongue of the patient, as he was accustomed to do upon such occasions, to ascertain the degree of animal temperature, with a view to future comparison. The paralytic man, wholly ignorant of the nature of the process to which he was to submit, but deeply impressed from the representation of Dr. Beddoes with the certainty of its success, no sooner felt the thermometer under his tongue than he concluded the talisman was in full operation, and in a burst of enthusiasm declared that he already experienced the effect of its benign influence through his whole body. The opportunity was too tempting to be lost; Davy cast one intelligent glance at Coleridge, and desired his patient to renew his visit the following day, when the same ceremony was performed, and repeated every succeeding day for a fortnight; the patient gradually improving during that period, when he was dismissed as cured, no other application having been used."

In a recent number of the *British Medical Journal* * some interesting observations are given from the *Student's Journal*, of the impressions which patients occasionally derive from the use of the clinical thermometer; a young woman who was convalescent, and whose temperature had long remained normal, had a slight relapse, which she attributed to having had "no glass under her arm for a week." A man suffering from acute rheumatism, obstinately refused to have his temperature taken any more, saying "it took too much out of him; it was

* January 29, 1876.

a drawing all his strength away." A man had been in the habit for some time of having his temperature taken daily under his tongue, with a thermometer that had just been doing severe duty in the axillæ of other patients. One night a bran new thermometer was applied to his mouth; next day he declared he was not so well, and said, "the glass was not so strong as usual; he felt at the time the taste was different, and it had not done him so much good." A sister in one of the woman's wards says, that many of the patients think the thermometers are used to detect breaches of the rule against having unauthorized edibles brought in by friends; and she, accordingly, does not disabuse their minds of their innocent superstition. These "impressions" are precisely the sort of evidence on which "metallic tractors," galvanic belts, mesmerists, and animal magnetisers rely for their vogue.

Only a few days ago a lady consulted me for a severe neuralgic attack, involving the fifth pair of nerves throughout one side of her face. In order to determine the relative temperature of the two sides, I applied to each cheek a thermo-electric pile in connection with a delicate galvanometer. Of course there was no sensation given to her beyond that of contact with the two little piles, but looking at the galvanometer, as it stood on the table she saw the deflection of the needle, and imagining that it was for the purpose of cure, exclaimed that she felt decidedly better, and expressed the belief that another application would entirely cure her. I again put the piles on her cheeks, with the result of completely relieving her of a pain with which she had suffered for five days.

Similar cases are common enough in the practice of all

physicians, and wise members of the profession taking them at their full value, can meditate on the problem which will continually recur to their minds: how much such a curative power, in any case, is to be ascribed to the purely medical treatment, and how much to that confidence in themselves, which, it should be no small part of their duty to endeavor to inspire by all honorable means, in the minds of those who put health and life in their hands. It is certainly true that the only advantage the charlatan has is his unscrupulousness; and this in the long run will probably bring him to grief. The educated physician, however, skilled as he should be in the working of the human mind, may, without the sacrifice of dignity or truth, avail himself of all the power which his knowledge gives him, and if he has reason to think, after a careful study of his patients' mental organization and disease, that colored water will probably effect the cure, it is his duty to use it, instead of resorting to medicines which, like a two-edged sword, may cut two ways at once.

CHAPTER XI.

PNEUMATOGRAPHIC AND WRITING MEDIUMS

A PNEUMATOGRAPHIC medium is one who is able to obtain writing direct from the spirits without the employment of any material agency. A writing medium is one of whom the spirits make use as a means of communication with human beings. According to Kardec the first are exceedingly rare, but are probably developed by exercise. When found, all that they have to do is to place paper in any spot designated by the spirits, to leave it there a few minutes, and then, on inspection, the spiritual message will be found written on it. Prayer and meditation are necessary adjuncts, and for that reason favorable results are impossible of attainment in a company of frivolous and scoffing people—not actuated by sympathetic and benevolent sentiments.

Ordinary writing mediums are quite common. As Kardec says, of all means of communication from spirits to human beings, writing is the most simple, the most convenient and the most complete. He might have added that of all methods it is the easiest for perpetrating fraud. All that a writing medium has to do is to take a pen in his hand, write what he chooses, and tells his dupes it comes from some spirit. There will always be idiots enough to believe him.

Both pneumatographic and writing mediumship afford such palpable opportunities for frauds that it is scarcely necessary to pursue this division of the subject further.

Somnambulistic, possessed and obsessed mediums, will be more appropriately considered under the heads to which the attention of the reader will next be invited.

CHAPTER XII.

SOMNAMBULISM—NATURAL AND ARTIFICIAL.

IN the condition known as somnambulism there appears to be a more or less perfect state of automatism, which is the governing power of the individual. Certain faculties and senses are intensely exalted, while others are as completely suspended in action. If the attention can be concentrated upon any particular idea, circumstance or object, great lucidity is manifested. On the other hand there may be, and generally is, the most profound abstraction of mind in regard to all other ideas and things.

The most thorough work on natural somnambulism, is that of Bertrand,* published over fifty years ago, but which is still admirable for the truthful account of the various phenomena attendant upon the condition in question. Bertrand assigns somnambulism to four causes:—

1. A particular nervous temperament, which predisposes individuals otherwise in good health to paroxysms of somnambulism during their ordinary sleep.

2. It is sometimes produced in the course of certain diseases, of which it may be considered a symptom or a crisis.

* "Traité du somnambulisme et des différentes modifications qu'il présente." Paris, 1823.

3. It is often seen in the course of the proceeding neces sary to bring on the condition known as animal magnetism.

4. It may result as a consequence of a high degree of mental exaltation. It is in this state contagious by imitation to such persons as are submitted to the same influence.

From these four categories of causes, Bertrand distinguishes four kinds of somnambulism—the natural, the symptomatic, the artificial, and the ecstatic. Under the artificial variety we must include Mr. Braid's hypnotism. In general terms, therefore, there are two kinds of somnambulism, the natural and the artificial. As an instance of the former condition, the following case is adduced from a recent monograph of the writer: *

"A young lady of great personal attractions had the misfortune to lose her mother by death from cholera. Several other members of the family suffered from the disease, she alone escaping, though almost worn out with fatigue, excitement, and grief. A year after these events her father removed from the West to New York, bringing her with him and putting her at the head of his household. She had not been long in New York before she became affected with symptoms resembling those met with in chorea. The muscles of the face were in almost constant action; and though she had not altogether lost the power to control them by her will, it was difficult at times for her to do so. She soon began to talk in her sleep, and finally was found one night by her father, as he came home, endeavoring to open the street door. She was then, as he said, sound asleep, and had to be violently shaken to be aroused. After this she made the attempt every night to get

* "Sleep and its Derangements," p. 205. Philadelphia, 1869.

out of bed, but was generally prevented by a nurse who slept in the same room with her, and who was awakened by the noise she made. Her father now consulted me in regard to the case, and invited me to the house in order to witness the somnambulic acts for myself. One night, therefore, I went to his residence, and waited for the expected manifestations. The nurse had received orders not to interfere with her charge on this occasion, unless it was evident that injury would result, and to notify us of the beginning of the performance.

"About twelve o'clock she came down stairs and informed us that the young lady had risen from her bed and was about to dress herself. I went up-stairs, accompanied by her father, and met her in the upper hall partly dressed. She was walking very slowly and deliberately, her head elevated, her eyes open, and her hands hanging loosely by her side. We stood aside to let her pass. Without noticing us, she descended the stairs to the parlor, we following her. Taking a match which she had brought with her from her own room, she rubbed it several times on the under side of the mantel-piece until it caught fire, and then, turning on the gas, lit it. She next threw herself into an arm-chair and looked fixedly at a portrait of her mother which hung over the mantel-piece. While she was in this position I carefully examined her countenance, and performed several experiments, with the view of ascertaining the condition of the senses as to activity.

"She was very pale, more so than was natural to her; her eyes were wide open, and did not wink when the hand was brought suddenly in close proximity to them; the muscles of the face, which, when she was awake, were almost constantly in action, were now perfectly still; her pulse was regular in rhythm and force, and beat eighty-two per minute, and the respiration was uniform and slow.

'I held a large book between her eyes and the picture she was apparently looking at, so that she could not see it. She nevertheless continued to gaze in the same direction as if no obstacle were interposed. I then made several motions as if about to strike her in the face. She made no attempt to ward off the blows, nor did she give the slightest sign that she saw my actions. I touched the corner of each eye with a lead-pencil I had in my hand, but even this did not make her close her eyelids. I was entirely satisfied that she did not see, at least with her eyes.

"I held a lighted sulphur-match under her nose, so that she could not avoid inhaling the sulphurous acid gas which escaped. She gave no evidence of feeling any irritation. Cologne-water and other perfumes and smelling-salts likewise failed to make any obvious impression on her olfactory nerves.

"Through her partially-opened mouth I introduced a piece of bread soaked in lemon-juice. She evidently failed to perceive the sour taste. Another piece of bread saturated with a solution of quinine was equally ineffectual. The two pieces remained in her mouth a full minute and were then chewed and swallowed.

"She now arose from her chair and began to pace the room in an agitated manner; she wrung her hands, sobbed, and wept violently. While she was acting in this way, I struck two books together several times so as to make loud noises close to her ears. This failed to interrupt her.

"I then took her by the hand and led her back to the chair in which she had previously been sitting. She made no resistance, but sat down quietly and soon became perfectly calm.

"Scratching the back of her hand with a pin, pulling her hair, and pinching her face, appeared to excite no sensation.

"I then took off her slippers and tickled the soles of her feet. She at once drew them away, but no laughter was produced. As often as this experiment was repeated, the feet were drawn up. The spinal cord was therefore awake.

"She had now been down-stairs about twenty minutes. Desiring to awake her, I shook her by the shoulders quite violently for several seconds without success.

I then took her head between my hands and shook it. This proved effectual in a little while. She awoke suddenly, looked around her for an instant, as if endeavoring to comprehend her situation, and then burst into a fit of hysterical sobbing. When she recovered her equanimity she had no recollection of any thing that had passed, or of having had a dream of any kind."

This case illustrates very well some of the principal phenomena of natural somnambulism. Many others are on record which, in many respects, are more remarkable, but it is scarcely necessary to refer to them here at greater length, though a word or two in regard to Jane Rider, the Springfield somnambulist, will be both instructive and interesting.

When she began her manifestations Jane Rider was in her seventeenth year. She was intelligent, of mild and obliging disposition, and had the confidence and esteem of those who knew her. Her education was superior to that of persons occupying her class in society, and she was particularly fond of poetry and of reading generally. She was of full habit and of prepossessing appearance, but was subject to headaches, and about three years previously was affected for several months with chorea. A small spot on the left side of her head had been tender from her earliest recollection, and the sensibility was much increased when she suffered from headache.

Dr. Belden,* from whose account I derive the foregoing and the following particulars, states that the first attack began on the night of June 24, 1832. When he saw her she was struggling to get out of bed, and complained at the same time of pain in the left side of the head. Her head was hot, the face flushed and her pulse much excited. An emetic was given her, and she vomited a large quantity of green currants; after which she became quiet.

Nearly a month elapsed before she had another paroxysm. Then, after several attempts on the part of her friends to keep her in bed, it was determined to allow her to take her own course and to watch her movements. Having dressed herself she went down stairs and proceeded to make preparations for breakfast. She set the table, arranged the various articles with the utmost precision, went into a dark room and into a closet at the most remote corner, from which she took the coffee cups, placed them on a waiter, turned it sideways to pass through the doors, avoided all intervening obstacles, and deposited the whole safely on the table.

She then went into the pantry, the blinds of which were shut, and the door closed after her. She then skimmed the milk, poured the cream into one cup and the milk into another without spilling a drop. She then cut the bread, placed it reg-

* An account of Jane C. Rider, the Springfield Somnambulist. Springfield, 1834.

ularly on the plate, and divided the slices in the middle. In fine, she went through the whole operation with as much precision as the cook in open day; and this with her eyes closed and without any light except that from one lamp which was standing in the breakfast room to enable the family to observe her operations. During the whole time, she seemed to take no notice of those around her, unless they purposely stood in her way, or placed chairs or other obstacles before her, when she avoided them, with an expression of impatience at being thus disturbed.

She finally returned voluntarily to bed, and on finding the table arranged for breakfast when she made her appearance in the morning, inquired why she had been allowed to sleep while another performed her work. None of the transactions of the preceding night had left the slightest impression on her mind.

Then she had many more paroxysms similar in general character to that just described, and during which she was submitted by Dr. Belden and others to many experiments. Though it was found that her sense of sight was greatly increased in acuteness, she had no clairvoyance, properly so-called. It was ascertained, too, that though she had no recollection, when awake, of what she had done during a paroxysm, she remembered in one paroxysm the events of the preceding one. Finally she was sent to the hospital at Worcester, and there, under suitable treatment, her seizures became less frequent and finally disappeared altogether.

Now, it has long been known that somnambulism can be artificially induced. Even before the time of Mesmer there were occasional illustrations of this fact; but Puysegur is entitled to the credit of being the first to systematize them and to practise the art of producing factitious somnambulism. He caused it by passes, and finally, it is claimed, by simple acts of the will. The Abbé Faria induced it by shouting, and Barberin by praying! Other methods were also employed; and, as its identity with mesmerism became generally recognized, it had ascribed to it the name of mesmeric or magnetic sleep.

No one has more thoroughly investigated the nature of artificial somnambulism than Mr. Braid,* who gives the following as his ordinary method of procedure:

"Take any bright object (I generally use my lancet-case) between the thumb and fore and middle fingers of the left hand, hold it from eight to fifteen inches from the eyes at such position above the forehead as may be necessary to produce the greatest possible strain upon the eyes and eyelids, and enable the patient to maintain a steady, fixed stare at the object. It will generally be found that the eyelids close with a *vibratory* motion, or become spasmodically closed. After ten or fifteen seconds have elapsed, by gently elevating the arms and legs, it will be found that the patient has a disposition to retain them in the situation in which they have been placed, if he is intensely affected. If this is not the case, desire him to retain the limbs in the extended position, and thus the pulse will speedily become greatly accelerated, and the limbs, in process of time, become quite rigid and involuntarily fixed. It will also be found that all the organs of special sense, excepting sight, including heat, and cold, and muscular motion or resistance, are *at first* prodigiously *exalted*, such as happens with regard to the primary effects of opium,

* "Neurypnology, or the Rationale of Nervous Sleep, considered in Relation with Animal Magnetism," etc. London, 1843.

wine, and spirits. After a certain point, however, this exaltation of function is followed by a state of depression far greater than the torpor of *natural* sleep. From the state of the most profound torpor of the organs of special sense and tonic rigidity of the muscles, they may at this stage *instantly* be restored to the *opposite* condition of extreme mobility and exalted sensibility, by directing a current of air against the organ or organs we wish to excite to action, or the muscles we wish to render limber, and which had been in this catalептiform state. By mere repose the senses will speedily merge into the original condition again."

Mr. Braid gives examples of this artificial somnambulism or hypnotism, as he designates it, which show that its phenomena are identical with those of natural somnambulism, and that it covers much that is alleged to be due to animal magnetism and modern spiritualism. He found the same condition to be produced, though he left the room, if the subject followed his directions, so that there could be no suspicion that he acted through the medium of any force emanating from his body.

The persons who most readily come into the hypnotic condition are of the same class as those who were such favorable subjects for the odic force of Von Reichenbach, and who now make the best mediums. The writer has very carefully investigated this division of the subject, and has made many experiments in regard to it, which leave no doubt in his mind that the relation really exists. As an illustration of the character of the phenomena, the following case is adduced. He does not doubt that the thoughtful reader will at once see, that if such a person, as the one whose actions while in the hypnotic state are described, should be disposed to deceive, or should be under the control of designing or ignorant individuals, she would not fail to be received by many as a medium of the first order.

A short time after writing the account of the young lady whose case has just been quoted as an example of natural somnambulism, I was informed by her father that her affection, which had been cured by suitable medical treatment, had returned, owing, as he supposed, to excessive mental exertion, she having contracted a taste for philosophy, in the study of which she had indulged to a great extent.

Upon examination, I found that she not only had paroxysms of natural somnambulism, but that she had acquired the power of inducing the hypnotic state at will. Her process was to take up some one of the philosophical works she was in the habit of studying, select a paragraph which required intense thought or excited powerful emotion, read it, close the book, fix her eyes steadily, but not directing the foci so as to see any particular object, and then reflect deeply upon what she had read. From the revery thus occasioned, she gradually passed into the somnambulic condition. During this state it was said she answered questions correctly, read books held behind her, described scenes passing in distant places, and communicated messages from the dead. She therefore possessed, in every essential respect, the qualifications of either a clairvoyant or a spiritualistic medium, according to the peculiar tenets of belief held by the faithful.

In accordance with my request, she proceeded to put herself into the hypnotic state. With a volume of Plato in her hand, she read thus from the Apology of Socrates. Her voice was calm and impressive, as though she felt every word she uttered:

"Moreover, we may hence conclude that there is great hope that death is a blessing. For to die is one of two things: for either the dead may be annihilated and have no sensation of any thing whatever, or, as it is said, there is a certain change and passage of the soul from one place to another. And if it is a privation of all sensation, as it were a sleep in which the sleeper has no dream, death would be a wonderful gain. For I think that if any one having selected a night in which he slept so soundly as not to have had a dream, and having compared this night with all the other nights and days of his life, should be required on consideration to say how many days and nights he had passed better and more pleasantly than this night throughout his life, I think that not only a private person, but even the great king himself, would find them easy to number in comparison with other days and nights. If, therefore, death is a thing of this kind, I say it is a gain; for thus all futurity appears to be nothing more than one night."

As she reached the close, her voice became inexpressibly sad, the book dropped from her hand, her eyes were fixed on vacancy, her hands lay quietly in her lap, her breath came irregularly, and tears were flowing down her cheeks. Her pulse, which before she began to read was eighty-four per minute, was now one hundred and eight. As her abstraction became more profound, it fell, till, when she was unconscious, three minutes after she ceased reading, it was only seventy-two.

To satisfy myself that she was completely hypnotized, I

held a bottle of strong *aqua ammoniæ* to her nostrils. She did not evince the slightest degree of sensibility. Touching the eye with the finger—a test that a person practising deception could not have borne—equally failed to afford the least response indicative of sensation. I was, therefore, satisfied that she was in the condition of artificial somnambulism.

To describe in detail all that took place would lengthen unduly this account; such parts, therefore, as are material, and which illustrate essential points, will alone be given.

The writer asked her if there were any spirits in the room.

"Yes."

"Whose spirits are they?"

"The spirit of Socrates is here, the spirit of Plato, the spirit of Schleiermacher." (She had been reading before my arrival "Schleiermacher's Introductions to the Dialogues of Plato.")

"Do you not also see the spirit of Schenkelfürst?"

This was a *ruse*, there being no such person.

"Schenkelfürst?" she asked.

"Yes; he was Schleiermacher's constant companion and friend."

"Schenkelfürst," she repeated; "what a singular name!"

She was silent for a moment, and then her face was lit up with a smile, and she exclaimed:

"I see him; he is a small, dark man, with sharp, piercing eyes; he wears a coat trimmed with fur; he approaches Schleiermacher; they embrace; they are talking to each other."

"Will not Schleiermacher send some message through you?"

"No; he has gone away with his friend."

"Will no other spirit communicate?"

"Yes, there is one coming now; a man with a mournful face; his name is Bruno—Giordano Bruno. He speaks; he says, 'O my friends, be of good cheer; there is no end, even as there has been no beginning; the weak-hearted fall from the ranks, and, for a time, are lost; but, as there is a portion of the divinity in all God's creatures, even they are regenerated.'"

She stopped, and then in a low voice said, while tears streamed down her cheeks:

"*Majori forsitan cum timore sententiam in me fertis quam ego accipiam*"—the words used by Bruno when sentence of death was pronounced upon him. She had finished reading his life a few weeks before.

Desiring to change the current of her thoughts, and also to test her powers of prevision, she was asked who would be the first patient to enter the office of the writer that day week, and with what disease would he or she be affected?

She answered promptly:

"A gentleman from Albany, I see him now; he is thin, and pale, and very weak; he is lame, I think he is paralyzed."

The first person in reality who entered the office on the day in question was a lady of New York, suffering from nervous headache.

She was then asked where her father was at that moment (4.10 P. M.). Her answer was: "At the corner of Wall Street and Broadway; he is looking at the clock on Trinity Church; he is waiting for a stage." During the hour between four o'clock and five her father was in Brooklyn.

A table with paper was now placed before her, a pencil put into her hand, and she was requested again to place herself *en rapport* with some spirit. She immediately began to write as follows: "Let all the world hear my voice and follow the precepts I inculcate. There are many fools and but few wise. I write for the former, and am probably a fool myself, for I constantly see a chasm yawning at my side; and though my intellect tells me there is no chasm near me, I place a screen so that I cannot see it. PASCAL." She had that very day been reading a memoir of Pascal, in which the hallucination referred to was mentioned.

The following conversation then took place:

"Where are you now?"

"In New York."

"No, you are in a vessel at sea; there is a terrible storm; are you not afraid?"

"Yes, I am very much frightened; what shall I do? Oh, save me, save me!"

She wrung her hands, screamed with terror, rose from her chair and paced the room, apparently suffering intensely from fear. In the midst of her agitation she awoke, and it was not without difficulty that the impression she had received could be removed.

On a subsequent occasion her somnambulic powers of vision were tested by asking her to read the writing on a slip of paper; to tell the time marked by a watch held to the back of her head; to read a particular line from a closed book, etc.; but, though she always made some answer, she was never once right. The senses of touch and of hearing were the only ones she appeared to be capable of exercising, and these were not in any degree exalted in their action. Conjoined with integrity of touch there was well-marked *analgesia*, or inability to feel pain. Thus, though able to tell the shape, texture, and consistence of objects placed in her hands, she experienced no sensation when a pin was thrust into the calf of her leg, or when a coal of fire was held in close proximity to any part of her body.

It will readily be preceived, therefore, that certain parts of her nervous system were in a state of inaction, were in fact dormant, while others remained capable of receiving sensations and originating nervous influence. Her sleep was therefore incomplete. Images were formed, hallucinations entertained, and she was accordingly in these respects in a condition similar to that of a dreaming person; for the images and hallucinations were either directly connected with thoughts she had previously had, or were immediately suggested to her through her sense of hearing. Some mental faculties were exercised, while others were quiescent. There was no correct judgment and no volition. Imagination, memory, the emotions, and *the ability to be impressed by suggestions*, were present in a high degree.

Now, the writer is satisfied, from a careful study of this lady's case, and of others similar to it in general character which have come under his observation, that the phenomena of hypnotism are not those of pure somnambulism, but that three other conditions are present in greater or less degree. These are hysteria, catalepsy, and ecstasy. To a brief consideration of some of the more important features of these abnormal states of the nervous system the attention of the reader will presently be invited.

That many of the phenomena exhibited by honest mediums are referable to the condition now under notice is not a matter for doubt; and this view is rendered still stronger by a consideration of the fact that the hypnotic state can be readily induced in many species of animals. This has been known, with different interpretations of the cause and nature of the condition, for very many years, but for a revival of the knowledge, and for giving incentives to new lines of inquiry, we owe a debt to the students of animal magnetism or mesmerism.

In 1646, Kircher, a Jesuit priest, and like many others of his fraternity, fond of scientific investigations, published an account of an experiment performed by him and which he called "*experimentum mirabile de imaginatione gallinæ*—a wonderful experiment showing the imagination of the hen.

He tied the hen's feet together with a cord, and then laid the animal on the ground, where, after struggling for a while, it lay perfectly quiet, as if despairing of escape, it had yielded to the superior will and power of its conqueror. Then with a piece of chalk Kircher drew two lines on the ground, one from each eye, and uniting at an acute angle a little in front of the head. He then loosened the band which fastened the legs together; but the hen, though physically free to escape, remained still, and could scarcely be forced out of its position.

So far, the facts; now for the theory. Kircher attributes this very remarkable result to the strong imaginative powers, with which, in his opinion, hens are gifted; for the animal seeing the chalk line, takes it for the string with which it had been fastened, and having acquired experience of the futility of all efforts to escape, and thinking itself still bound, remains perfectly quiet on the ground.

The late Prof. Czermak, a short time before his death, placed Kircher's and similar experiments before the world in their true light; and I therefore do not hesitate to cite his observations at some length.*

While on a visit to Bohemia, Czermak was informed, by a gentleman whose acquaintance he made, that he had not only seen crawfish magnetized, but had himself put these animals into the magnetic state, and that the matter was exceedingly simple.

The crawfish is to be held firmly in one hand, while with the other, passes are to be made from the tail of the animal towards the head. Under this manifestation the crawfish now becomes quiet, and if placed on its head in a vertical position, remains motionless until passes are made in the opposite direction, when it staggers, falls, and finally crawls away.

Czermak did not question the facts, but he doubted the explanation and expressed a desire to witness the experiment. A basket of crawfish was obtained from a neighboring brook, and the friend, sure of his results, seized one of the animals and began his "magnetic strokes" from the tail to the head. The crawfish, which at first resisted, gradually became calm, and finally stood erect on its head, remaining motionless as if

* Czermak's experiments were performed before the class of the private physiological laboratory of the University of Leipsic, Jan. 24th and 25th, 1873, and were published with his remarks in subsequent numbers of the "*Gartenlaube.*" These lectures were translated by Clara Hammond and published in the "*Popular Science Monthly,*" Sept. and Nov., 1873.

asleep, in this forced and unnatural position, supporting itself with its antennæ and two under claws.

But in the mean time Czermak had taken one of the crawfish and endeavored to make it stand on its head without the passes being previously made. The animal staggered at first, as did the other, and ended by becoming perfectly quiet and standing on its head exactly as had the one which had been magnetized.

As to the awakening process the friend made his passes from the head to the tail and Czermak made his from the tail to the head. The result was the same in both, for both soon fell over and crawled away. In fact whether the strokes were made or not, the animals regained their normal condition in about the same length of time.

Hence it was demonstrated that "magnetic passes" were neither necessary to induce the hypnotic state nor to cause the animal to emerge from it. The act, therefore, constituted what Czermak calls "a fact viewed unequally." His friend had not thoroughly investigated the phenomenon in all its relations, and that is just what is done every day by certain people calling themselves "inquirers," who make imperfect attempts to solve the pseudo-mysteries of mesmerism, spiritualism, etc.

Now to return to Kircher and his experiments, which he thought demonstrated the existence of a great degree of imagination in the hen.

It has long been known that wild and frightened hens may be rendered perfectly quiet by placing them, for instance, on a table and holding them there while a chalk line is drawn so as to connect the eyes; or even a single line for an inch or two from the end of the beak. In calling attention to this fact Czermak caused one of his assistants to bring him a hen and to hold it fast on the table. This was done after much resistance and many cries from the frightened bird. Then, with his left hand he held the head and neck of the hen upon the table, and with his right hand drew a chalk line on the table, beginning at the end of the beak. Left entirely free, the hen, though breathing heavily, remained entirely quiet on the table; then without resistance it allowed itself to be placed on its back, in which unnatural position it remained till the end of the lecture, not awaking till the audience began to leave.

Czermak states that when he first performed this experiment, he was for a moment dumb with astonishment, for the hen not only remained motionless in its forced and unnatural position, but did not make the slightest attempt to fly away or to move in any manner when he endeavored to startle it. It was clear that the hen had altogether lost the functional capacities of its nervous system, under the apparently indifferent and useless arrangements of the experiment, and had placed herself in this remarkable condition as though by magic. But Czermak was not a man to stand still at an "event viewed unequally," and as soon as he recovered from his extreme astonishment at the result, he rubbed out the chalk line. The hen still remained perfectly quiet. But as this might have been due to the continuing effect of the chalk line, he performed another experiment in which he held the hen firmly for some time and stretched out the head and neck as though he were going to draw the chalk line, but in reality he did not draw it. He then released the hen and the animal remained just as immovable as in the previous experiment.

The cord around the legs and the chalk line were therefore entirely unnecessary, and accordingly Kircher's theory of the imagination of the hen falls to the ground. The only part which survives is the immobility of the hen when laid upon a table after having been previously held in the hand for a short time. He has therefore reported an unequally viewed event. He stopped too soon in his investigations, and in his anxiety to discover a cause for the remarkable phenomenon before him, jumped at a conclusion which, as we have seen, has nothing whatever to support it. Suppose Mr. Crookes or Mr. Wallace had seen Mr. Home perform this experiment, and that they had never heard of it before. Can there be a doubt that had he told them that the hen was held down by the power of a spirit they would have been ready to believe him ? This is exactly what they have done in accepting his theories of levitation, immunity from fire, accordeon playing, raising weights, etc.

I have repeatedly performed Czermak's experiments, using young lobsters, frogs, hens, geese and ducks, with scarcely a failure. Of all animals in my experience, the frog passes into the hypnotic condition most readily. All that is necessary is to hold it firmly for a minute or two by the sides of the body just behind the fore legs, and then gently lay it on its back on a table, board, or palm of the hand. So profound is the hypnotism that the blade of a pair of scissors may be introduced into the lower part of the belly and the animal cut open its whole length, without its moving, or apparently experiencing the least sensation. Over ten years ago I became acquainted with the possibility of inducing the condition in question in frogs, and often in my medical lectures brought the fact before the class in attendance. In general, without the causation of hypnotism, there is no position seemingly so disagreeable to a frog as the dorsal, and it gets out of it as soon as possible.

But with some animals it appears as if an object to gaze at is necessary in order to produce the hypnotic state, and hence we cannot say that the chalk line of Kircher, or something analogous is in every case unnecessary. Thus pigeons are not brought into this condition by simply stretching out their necks and holding them firmly for a short time. Czermak ascertained that in order to hypnotize them it was requisite to hold something, as the finger, before their eyes, so as to attract their attention, and then the birds remained rigid and motionless as if tired, for several minutes. The same result follows if a piece of glass tube, a cork, a small wax candle, or any other equally lifeless object, be placed on the top of the pigeon's bill. All that is necessary, is to place the article in such a position as to admit of its attention being attracted and fixed upon the substance used.

And with hens; if they be seized by the bodies with both hands so that their heads and necks are quite free, and the bodies be pressed against a pedestal on which a glass tube rests so as to come in contact with their bills, they remain perfectly quiet for some time gazing at the object before them.

Again, if a piece of twine be hung so that the end comes just between the eyes, a hen not only remains perfectly motionless but closes its eyes and sleeps, the head sinking till it comes in contact with the table. Before falling asleep, the hen's head can be pressed down or raised up and it will remain in the position in which it may be placed, as though it were made of wax. This fact shows the analogy which exists between hypnotism and catalepsy as it occurs in the human subject, and to which attention will presently be invited.

In this connection I may state that I have recently repeated an experiment which I remember to have seen when a boy, long before Mr. Braid began his investigations, and which shows that there is at least one other way of inducing hypnotism in hens. I took a hen, and putting its head under its wing, held it in that position for a couple of minutes. On placing it on a table, it stood erect without removing its head from the position in which I had placed it, and remained motionless for several minutes apparently in a deep sleep. As I had formerly seen this experiment, it was somewhat different. The head was placed under the wing, and then the animal, held in that position, was swung round three or four times before being placed on the ground. The explanations then given of the subsequent insensibility was, that the animal was affected with vertigo, and did not move for fear of falling.

Czermak therefore found, as he proceeded with his investigations, that the drawing of the chalk line in Kircher's experiment was of some significance, though not such as the old priest supposed. The hand which draws the line, and the line itself constitute an object upon which the animal's look and attention are placed, and there is developed a marvellous condition of certain parts of its nervous system, accompanied by cataleptic phenomena and sleep.

We have already seen how Mr. Braid produced hypnotism in the human subject, and we now perceive that a like process causes it in the lower animals.

Upon one occasion Mr. Braid, in the presence of eight hundred persons, put ten full grown men, out of fourteen, into a state of complete sleep; all began the experiment at the same time. The persons fixed their eyes steadily upon pieces of cork fastened upon their foreheads; the others of their own will gazed steadily at certain points in the direction of the audience. In three minutes the eyelids of the ten had involuntarily closed. With some, consciousness remained; others were cataleptic and entirely insensible to being stuck with needles, and others on awaking knew absolutely nothing of what had taken place during their sleep. In 1859, Velpeau and Broca, two distinguished French surgeons, placed twenty-four women in the hypnotic condition by Braid's method, and then performed surgical operations on them without causing the slightest pain.

I have repeatedly placed women in the hypnotic state, and performed surgical operations which would otherwise have caused great pain, without the least sensation having been experienced. Only a few days ago I cauterized, with a red-hot iron, the spine of a lady, having previously hypnotized her by causing her to look for a few minutes at a cork which I had fastened to her forehead a little above the root of the nose. The anæsthesia was complete, and the sleep so profound that she not only did not hear the sound produced by the burning of the skin, but very loud noises made close to her ears were equally unperceived. After about seven minutes she spontaneously awoke.

Czermak was preparing to extend his observations to mammals, but death prevented the fulfilment of his intentions. Experiments of my own, however, show that there is no difficulty in bringing dogs, rabbits, and cats fully under the hypnotic influence. Rabbits require to be held firmly in the hands at the same time that some bright object, as a key, is allowed to hang from a string, just in front of, and a little above the eyes. Five or at most ten minutes are sufficient to induce hypnotism.

Or, the animal may be held firmly in a squatting position on a table while an object, as a key, a piece of chalk, or a cork, is placed about an inch in front of its nose. After a few minutes sleep ensues.

With dogs, the procedure is much simpler. My experiments have been conducted with the several varieties that have been taught to stand up on their haunches and "beg." It is exceedingly easy to engage their attention and thus to cause them to pass into the hypnotic state. For this purpose a piece of chalk the size of a cherry is fastened to a string and allowed to hang between the eyes of the dog at a distance of an inch or two. The experiment seems to succeed better if the animal be made to take the begging position, though this is not necessary. Indeed, the condition can often be induced by simply engaging the attention of the dog for a few minutes by pointing the finger at him, or by any other convenient method.

After a due consideration of the experiments of Czermak and myself, we are able to appreciate, at their full value, the accounts which are given us of miraculous and mesmeric power exercised by man over the lower animals. Thus we may dismiss as absolutely untrue the stories which are told of the bees coming to Sts. Ambrose, Isidore, Dominic, and others, while they were yet infants, and depositing honey on their lips, and of following them into the desert and obeying the commands addressed to them. We may also refuse to regard as within the domain of truth, the account given of St. Rose of Lima by Görres,* as follows:

This young lady had built a little arbor in her mother's

* *Op., cit.*, t. 1, p. 480.

garden, and was accustomed to repair thither for meditation and praise. The place was continually thronged night and day by mosquitoes, the walls were covered with them, and the music of their hum continually resounded throughout the place. Not one of them, however, ever touched her, but if her mother or any other person visited her in her solitude they were at once bitten and their blood sucked by the insatiable insects. Every one was astonished that St. Rose was never injured by them. But she smiling, said "When I came here I made a pact with these little creatures." [It would have been somewhat more filial if she had included her mother in the bargain.] "It was agreed that they should not bite me and that I should not injure them. Therefore they dwell here in peace with me; and not only that, but they aid me with all their power to praise God." In fact every time the virgin came into the arbor at sunrise she said to the mosquitoes. "Come, my friends, let us praise God," and then the little insects formed a circle around her, and began their little songs with a degree of order and harmony such as no choir directed by a master could have excelled; and this was kept up until the saint enforced silence upon them.

These circumstances are cited by Pope Clement X. in the bull canonizing St. Rose.

It must be admitted that the character of the mosquito has greatly degenerated since that time, for it has, apparently, acquired habits of association with demons rather than saints.

Fish, reptiles, birds and mammals, have also been brought under saintly influence. Jacques de Cerqueto, an Augustine monk, enforced silence on the frogs that troubled him when he was saying mass. St. Ida could not approach a stream without hundreds of fish coming to greet her, and if she placed her hands in the water, "the fish took hold of her fingers as infants do the breasts of their mothers."

Gondisalvo Amaranthi, being in want one day of a dinner, made the sign of the cross on the river near by, and instantly numerous fish placed themselves at his disposal. The good man took what he wanted and put the rest back into the water. St. Joseph of Copertino, among others, controlled birds, making them sing when he wished, and St. Jacques de Stephano was thanked by a flock of pigeons which he had saved from destruction at the hands of some hunters.

Among quadrupeds, lions have always been remarkable for the docility with which they submit to saintly influence. From the time of Daniel, down through the early ages of Christianity, these naturally ferocious beasts have at times shown an appreciation of the character of those exposed to their fury, which is certainly not a usual attribute of their savage nature.

St. Thomas of Florence calmed furious bulls by a single word. St. Francis de Paul selected two of the most savage of these animals out of a herd and led them like lambs. The like is asserted of wild horses and angry dogs, both kinds of animals being quieted by a look, a word, or a gesture from a saint or other holy person.

It would scarcely be wise to refuse belief to all incidents of the kind which are referred to in the acts of the saints. We can accept some as being true in point of fact, and we attribute the result, not to supernatural agency, but to the hypnotic power, illustrations of which have engaged our attention.

Strange to say, however, the influence over the lower

animals is denied, or at least regarded by some mesmerists as not proven. Thus, Teste* states that the results are so vague, so fleeting, so inappreciable, that it is not possible to certify their existence.

But, on the other hand, Dr. Elliotson believes fully in the mesmeric power of man over the brute creation, and gives several instances in support of his opinions. Among them the following.† The Duke of Marlborough, writing to Dr. Elliotson, says:—

"At Lord Ely's farm there is a yard dog so savage and ferocious that no one can approach him. I was determined to beat him and in thirty minutes had him fast asleep, his last sigh being a deep growl. In presence of several persons I then kissed the dog on his forehead, and then left him to awake at his leisure."

A month afterwards the dog was still stupid.

Again the Duke wrote to Dr. Elliotson. "I must now tell you what I have been doing here. I have also a very savage yard dog, I tried him to-day; in about fifteen minutes he ran into his kennel and hid his eyes from the manipulating process growling, snarling, and biting most furiously; notwithstanding, I then made the man who feeds him, and who is the only person who dares go near him, drag him out of his kennel and nail up a hurdle before the entrance, so as to keep him effectually outside. I then went to work again, the dog, as you may suppose, being ten times more ferocious. In about five minutes

* "A Practical Manual of Animal Magnetism," etc., translated by D. Chillan, M.D., etc., London, 1843, p. 226.

† "Mesmeric Phenomena in Brutes; as effected by the Duke of Marlborough and the Rev. Mr. Bartlett," *Zoist*, October, 1850. p. 295.

I had him so quiet, oppressed and stupid, that he dropped his nose several times in the mud around his kennel. Carts and horses, and men and boys were passing and repassing, which served continually to alarm him, so that I could not satisfactorily complete the task and leave him dead asleep ; besides which a heavy snowstorm was falling all the while, and I could not feel my finger ends. But I completely subdued the beast and patted him on the head before I left."

The Rev. Mr. Bartlett writes as follows :

"Upon descending a mountain I found myself in a narrow road between two stone fences which perhaps separated the lands of different proprietors. On one side of the fences were cattle and a bull. The bull approached the fence in an angry mood and walked along the other side of it parallel with me for more than a quarter of a mile : he then grew more excited, tore the ground with his horns, and bellowed fiercely. As I could not but apprehend that, should there be a breach in the wall, he might leap over and attack me, I was considering what course it was best to take, when we came to a very high and strong gate. Upon reaching the gate the bull rushed close up to it and bellowed loudly through it. As I knew that he could neither leap over nor force this gate I also approached it and looked him steadily in the face. In about a minute I caught his eye, which then fixed upon me, in about another minute a trembling of the eyelids arose, very similar to that of a human subject at an early stage of mesmeric influence. After probably three or four minutes, the eyes gradually closed, and the bull remained quiet and appeared to be as immovable as if he had been chiseled by the hand of the sculptor. The transition from his previously excited state to that of his perfectly motionless state was indeed most striking.

"I could not but feel thankful that all danger from the bull was now passed and after looking at his fixed form for a few moments I descended the remainder of the mountain, and *did not stop to wake him.*"

That some animals possess the power of acting upon others so as to induce a condition analogous to, if not indentical with, hypnotism, is well known. Serpents appear to be especially endowed with this faculty, and make use of it to secure birds and mammals for food. There is some reason also for believing that serpents can, in rare cases, exercise a like influence over man.

Now, after this survey of some of the principal phenomena of natural and artificial somnambulism are we able to determine in what their condition essentially consists? I am afraid we shall be obliged to answer this question in the negative, and mainly for the reason, that with all the study which has been given to the subject, we are not yet sufficiently well acquainted with the normal functions of the nervous system to be in a position to pronounce with definiteness on their aberrations. Nevertheless, the matter is not one of which we are wholly ignorant. We have some important data upon which to base our investigations into the philosophy of the condition in question, and inquiry, even if leading to erroneous results, at least promotes reflection and discussion, and may in time carry us to absolute truth.

If we turn our attention to the operations of the mind—by which term I understand the force developed by nervous action—we shall see that they are performed under two very different conditions. In the one there is consciousness; in the other unconsciousness.

A few examples will place the matter more distinctly before the reader.

If we are engaged in composing or writing, the only part of the process of which we are conscious, is the conception of our ideas, or the expression of them in suitable language. We are not conscious of every motion we give the pen. We do not even think of it, our whole attention being engrossed with higher thoughts. We can turn our minds to the penmanship if we are so disposed, and can make it the chief subject of our thoughts; but persons who write out original ideas rarely bother themselves with the nice formation of the letters. Hence their handwriting is generally bad, in the ordinary sense of the term. On the other hand, persons who copy, or those whose writing is not the expression of much thought, usually write with care and precision; to do so, is with them the chief object.

Or in the act of walking: a person, for instance, desires to measure the length of a room by pacing it. He starts at one end of it and makes his steps, conscious of each one, for his attention is turned especially to them; he counts them, in fact, and when he gets to the end knows exactly what he has done from the beginning to the end. Another person rises from his chair for the purpose of going to the book-case for a volume he desires. His mind is not on his steps—his will is directed towards getting the book he wants. He goes to the place where he knows it to be, but is not conscious of the act or method of getting there; but his legs have been accurately directed, there has been no mistake, his feet have been raised at exactly the right moments, and obstacles in the way have been avoided.

At another time we may begin to wind our watch. At that very instant some engrossing subject comes to our mind, we lose all consciousness of the act we have set out to perform, and yet it is carried out to the end, the key is taken out, the watch is closed and put in its pocket, and we may go on and perform other movements to which we have been accustomed before consciousness takes cognizance of the actions. In fact, so thoroughly taken up is consciousness with the thoughts which have come into the mind, that it fails altogether, at times, to embrace within its scope the act of winding the watch; and hence we do not know whether we have performed the act or not, and we begin the whole movement over again.

Again, a person will play a difficult piece of music and carry on a conversation at the same time; the conversation, if more interesting, engrosses the consciousness, and the music is performed automatically or unconsciously. If the piece has not been thoroughly learned, mistakes are made. If, on the other hand, the music interests more than the conversation, the individual is *distrait* and errors are committed, which show that the thoughts are not in the speech.

It would be easy to adduce other familiar examples, but the intelligent reader will have many such occur to his or her mind as instances in daily, hourly experience.

Now, somnambulism, natural or artificial, appears to be a

condition in which consciousness is subordinated to automatism; the subject performs acts of which there is no complete consciousness, and often none at all. Consequently there is little or no subsequent recollection. There is diminished activity of those parts of the nervous system which preside over certain faculties of the mind, while those which are capable of acting automatically are unduly exalted in power.

The condition is therefore analogous to sleep; for in all sleep there is in reality something of somnambulism. For the higher mental organs, as the sleep is more or less profound, are more or less removed from the sphere of action, leaving to the others the duty of performing such acts as may be required, or even of initiating others not growing out of the immediate wants of the system. If this quiescent state of the brain is accompanied, as it often is in nervous and excitable persons, by an exalted condition of the spinal cord, we have the higher order of somnambulistic phenomena produced, such as walking, or the performance of complex and apparently systematic movements; if the sleep of the brain be somewhat less profound and the spinal cord less excitable, the somnambulic manifestations do not extend beyond sleep-talking; a still less degree of cerebral inaction and spinal irritability produces simply a restless sleep and a little muttering; and when the sleep is perfectly natural and the nervous system of the individual well balanced, the movements do not extend beyond changing the position of the head and limbs and turning over in bed.

But the actions of the spinal cord—which is, I conceive, the organ chiefly controlling the mind in somnambulism—are not always automatic in character, as I have endeavored to show in another place.* The motions of frogs and of some other animals when deprived of their brains exhibit a certain amount of intellection or volition. That they are not more extensive is probably due to the fact that all the organs of the senses except that of touch have been removed with the brain, and hence the mechanism for coming into relation with the external world is necessarily diminished.

In profound somnambulism the whole brain is probably in a state of complete sleep, the spinal cord alone being awake. In partial or incomplete somnambulistic conditions certain of the cerebral ganglia are not entirely inactive, and hence the individual answers questions, exhibits emotions, and is remarkably disposed to be affected by ideas suggested by others. The ability to originate trains of thought exists only in very imperfect somnambulistic states.

Thus a girl, just after her first communion, while impressed with the solemnity of the occasion, or with the conversation which had been addressed to her, fell into a somnambulistic state, and exclaimed that she saw beautiful and glorious things. When asked by the elders around her what she saw, she answered, "God surrounded by the angels, the apostles, and Mary." Subsequently this girl got into the company of an individual who was a great admirer of Voltaire, and others of his philosophical sect, and on one occasion was hypnotized by him. Again she saw glorious

* The Brain not the Sole Organ of the Mind.—*Journal of Nervous and*

sights, and when he asked her what she saw she replied, "God, accompanied by His two apostles, Voltaire and Rousseau." *

In this and similar cases the brain originates nothing. It simply reflects the ideas which have recently been brought prominently before it, just as in dreams we imagine things and events with which in our waking moments the attention has been engaged.

The existence of a tendency to natural somnambulism is evidence of a highly impassionable and irritable nervous organization. Young persons are more often its subjects than those of mature age, and there are few children, who do not exhibit, at some time or other, manifestations of the condition in question, such as muttering or talking in their sleep, laughing, crying, or getting out of bed. The same irritable nervous system leads often to the supervention of other conditions, more of the nature of actual disease, such as catalepsy, ecstasy, epilepsy, chorea, convulsion, tremor, etc.

Much may be done in the way of medical treatment to correct the faulty neurotic condition, and much also, which more properly lies within the domain of home management. The reading of exciting fictions, and the witnessing of sensational theatrical exhibitions, are always prejudicial to persons subject to attacks of somnambulism.

Somnambulism often exists in conjunction with other affec

* Franz Dilitzsch, D.D., Professor of Theology, Leipsic. A System of Biblical Psychology. Translated from the German, by the Rev. Robert Ernest Wallis, Ph.D. Second English Edition. Edinburgh, 1875, p. 367.

tions of the nervous system. Its relations to spiritualism have been pointed out in the foregoing pages. But the association with hysteria, catalepsy, ecstasy and other morbid conditions, is of great interest and will next engage our attention.

CHAPTER XIII.

HYSTERIA.

IT is not to be expected that, in a work like the present, hyster a can be treated with that degree of fulness requisite for the study of the disorder in all its multiform aspects; neither would that be desirable, as such a course would lead us far into the domain of pure medical science, and one object—the principal which I had in writing this little work, would be defeated. All that is necessary or proper, is to make the reader acquainted with certain broad features of the affection, and to indicate the relations which it bears to various delusions—spiritualism among them.*

There is a strong tendency in all persons afflicted with hysteria, to the occurrence of symptoms which simulate organic diseases of various kinds. Paralysis, both of motion and of sensation, is one of the morbid conditions thus assumed; this tendency is not generally voluntary, though undoubtedly cases are not infrequent in which the simulation is clearly intentional, and others more numerous, in which volition, when drought to bear with full force upon the disposition, will over-

* For a full account of hysteria and hysterical affections, the reader is referred to the author's treatise on Diseases of the Nervous System, sixth edition. New York, 1876.

come it. In these latter cases there is, as it were, a paralysis of the will. In other instances, hysterical persons will deliberately enter upon a systematic course of deception and fraud, more apparently for the sake of attracting attention and obtaining notoriety, than from any other motive.

Thus, a hysterical woman will suddenly take to her bed and declare that she has no feeling and no power in her arms or legs. The most careful examination shows that she is speaking the truth. Pins may be thrust into the affected limb, it may be punctured or scorched *ad libitum*, and yet the possessor does not wince. A somewhat analogous state exists in us all at times. When the mind is intensely occupied, or the passions greatly aroused, there is a like insensibility to pain. Many a soldier wounded in battle, has not discovered his injury till the heat of the contest was over. We have seen how a similar insensibility to pain, is present during the somnambulic or hypnotic condition.

Now, when great mental exaltation is induced in a hysterical person, we find this analgesic condition developed to its utmost extent. Under these combined influences weak girls have submitted to all kinds of maltreatment and suffered no pain, and have been able to resist blows and other bodily injuries, which in their normal condition would have caused death. Thus it is stated by Montgeron,* in his account of the Jansenist Convulsionnaires, who visited the tomb of the Abbé Paris, that some women gave themselves severe blows with iron instruments in such a manner, that sharp points were forced

* La Vérité des Miracles, tome ii. 1737. Quoted by Calmeil, De la Folie, etc. Paris, 1845.

into the flesh. Fouillon states that another had herself hung up by the heels with the head downward, and remained in this position three-quarters of an hour. One day as she lay extended on her bed, two men who held a cloth under her back, raised her up and threw her forward two thousand four hundred times, while two other persons placed in front, thrust her back. Another day, four men having taken hold of her by the extremities, began to pull her, each with all his strength, and she was thus dragged in different directions for the space of some minutes. She caused herself to be tied one day as she lay on the table, her arms crossed behind her back and her legs flexed to their fullest extent, and, while six men struck her without ceasing, a seventh choked her. After this she remained insensible for some time, and her tongue, inflamed and discolored, hung far out of her mouth. Another insisted upon receiving a hundred blows upon the stomach with an andiron, and these were so heavy that they shook the wall against which she was placed, and upon one occasion a breach in it was caused at the twenty-fifth blow.

A physician, hearing of these things, insisted that they could not be true, as it was physically impossible that the skin, the flesh, the bones, and the internal organs, could resist such violence. He was told to come and verify the facts. He hastened to do so, and was struck with astonishment. Scarcely believing his eyes, he begged to be allowed to administer the blows. A strong iron instrument, sharp at one end, was put into his hands; he struck with all his might and thrust it deep into the flesh, but the victim laughed at his efforts, and remarked that his blows only did her good.

The government tried for a long time, unsuccessfully, to stop the epidemic, and at last was obliged to close the tomb and to place a guard over it, with orders to disperse the crowd that habitually collected in the cemetery, and to arrest the convulsionnaires. A wit of the period was almost justified in sticking up the following lines over the gate :—

"De par le Roi, défense à Dieu
De faire miracle dans ce lieu."

"And," says Voltaire, who relates this event, "Ce qu'il y a de plus étonnant, c'est qui Dieu obéit."

This immunity from injury, though remarkable, is frequently met with among hysterical persons at the present day, but is much more frequently assumed. Calmeil* states that many of the Jansenist fanatics were subject to great illusions on this point ; for many among them exhibited very obvious effects of the treatment, such as patches of discoloration on the skin, and innumerable contusions on the parts which had suffered the most severe assaults. Then it must be remembered that the blows upon the belly were given while the paroxysms were present, and when the stomach and intestines were distended with wind—a condition almost inseparable from the hysterical state. The prize-fighters of our own day, by filling the chest with air, endure blows which untrained persons could not receive without serious injury.

The writer has had the opportunity of witnessing many manifestations of hysteria analogous in character to those described in the foregoing remarks. Upon one occasion, a young

* *Op. cit.*, tome ii. p. 386.

woman, a patient in the wards of the Pennsylvania Hospit began a series of movements consisting in bending her bo backward till it formed an arch, her heels and head alone re ing on the bed, and then, suddenly straightening herself o would fall heavily. Instantly the arch was formed agai again she fell; and this process was kept up with inconceival rapidity for several hours every day. In another instance lady, during an access of hysterical paroxysms to which s was liable, beat her head with such violence against a lath a plaster partition, that she made a hole in it, while little or injury was inflicted on herself. In another, a girl eighte years of age lay down on the floor, naked, and made all t members of her family, five in number, stand each in turn f several minutes on her abdomen. In another, a lady, in orc that she might resemble those martyrs who suffered on t rack, tied her wrists with a stout cord, mounted a step-ladd fastened the cord to a hook in the wall, and then, jumping frc the ladder, succeeded in dislocating her shoulder. In anoth a lady rigidly closed her mouth, and refused to open it, eith to take food or to speak, for over forty-eight hours. No for that it was safe to use, could overcome the contraction of h muscles, and no persuasion induce her to relax them. S only yielded to an irresistible impulse to talk, and a degree hunger that human nature could no longer endure. It wou be easy to go on and cite, from the writer's practice or frc monographs on the subject, hundreds of other instances hysterical folly in which the subjects have been able to viola the laws of their being without apparently suffering serio pain or injury.

During the sixteenth and seventeenth centuries, an epidemic of hysterical chorea with catalepsy prevailed in many convents of Europe, and many grievous wrongs were in consequence inflicted upon perfectly innocent persons whom the "possessed" accused of having bewitched them; among others, Louis Gaufridi, a priest of Marseilles, and a man of cultivation and strict morality, was accused by two Ursuline nuns, named Madeline de Mandol and Louise Capel, the latter but nineteen years of age. At the time of the accusation these women were suffering from attacks of a hysterical kind, accompanied with hallucinations and illusions, fearful convulsions and cataleptic paroxysms, all of which were ascribed to possession of the devil, moved and instigated by Louis Gaufridi. At first, the accused denied the charges made against him, and endeavored by arguments to show the true nature of the seizures. The effort was in vain; he became insane, and confessed all that was laid to his charge, with numerous other offences, which had not been imagined. He declared that he had worshipped the devil for fourteen years, and that "ce démon m'engagea à rendre amoureuses de ma personne toutes les femmes que j'atteindrais de mon souffle. Plus de mille femmes ont été empoisonnées par l'attrait irrésistible de mon sòuffle qui les rendraient passionnées. La dame de la Pallude, mère de Madeleine, a été prise pour moi d'un amour insensé et s'est abandonnée à moi soit au sabbat soit hors du sabbat."

Gaufridi was burned at the stake, and the two Ursuline nuns "continuerent à délirer." * Among the convents visited by this terrible disorder was that of Sainte-Brigitte, at Lille.

* Calmeil. De la Folie, etc. Paris, 1845, t. i., p. 489, *et seq.*

Several of the nuns had been present at the proceedings against Gaufridi, and had thus been subjected to influences readily capable of producing the disease.

Among the sisters was one named Marie de Sains, who was remarkable for her many virtues, but who was now suspected of devoting herself to sorcery and of being the cause of the "possessions" of which the other nuns were the victims. She remained a year in prison, without any formal proofs of her guilt being adduced, until at last she was positively accused by three of the sisters with having intercourse with demons. At first, the poor nun appeared to be surprised at this charge; but suddenly she recanted her denial, and avowed herself the perpetrator of a series of such wicked and abominable acts, that it was difficult to understand how the conception of them had ever entered her mind. Among them were numberless murders, stranglings of innocent children, ravaging of graves, feeding on human flesh, revelling in orgies of superhuman atrocity, unheard-of sacrileges, poisonings, and in fact every imaginable crime. In the presence of her accusers and exorcists she improvised sermons which she ascribed to Satan, discoursed learnedly on the apocalypse, and made long discourses on antichrist. Like others of the present day, she was a speaking medium.

Marie de Sains was not burnt. She was merely stripped of her religious character, and condemned to perpetual imprisonment at Tournay.

A more noted example of spiritual possession is that afforded by the nuns of Loudun, and which resulted in the death of Urban Grandier at the stake, after he had been submitted to the most atrocious tortures, in the vain attempt to make him confess to an alliance with the devil.*

As showing the nature of the phenomena exhibited in the cases of monomania occurring among the nuns of Loudun, the following questions were proposed by Santerre, priest and promoter of the diocese of Nîmes, to the University of Montpelier:

Question 1. Whether the bending, bowing, and removing of the body, the head touching sometimes the soles of the feet, with other contortions and strange postures, are a good sign of possession?

2. Whether the quickness of the motion of the head forward and backward, bringing it to the back and breast, be an infallible mark of possession?

3. Whether a sudden swelling of the tongue, the throat and the face, and the sudden alteration of the color, are certain marks of possession?

4. Whether dulness and senselessness, or the privation of sense, even to be pinched and pricked without complaining, without stirring, and even without changing color, are certain marks of possession?

5. Whether the immobility of all the body which happens to the pretended possessed, by the command of their exorcists, during and in the middle of the strongest agitations, is a certain sign of a truly diabolical possession?

* For a very full account of this lamentable event, see the "Cheats and Illusions of Romish Priests and Exorcists discovered in the History of the Devils of Loudun. Being an account of the Pretended Possession of the Ursuline Nuns, and of the Condemnation and Punishment of Urban Grandier, a Parson of the same town. London, 1705.

6. Whether the yelping or barking like that of a dog, in the breast rather than in the throat, is a mark of possession?

7. Whether a fixed, steady look upon some object, without moving the eye on either side, be a good mark of possession?

8. Whether the answers that the pretended possessed made in French, to some questions that are put to them in Latin, are a good mark of possession?

9. Whether to vomit such things as people have swallowed, be a sign of possession?

10. Whether the prickings of a lancet upon divers parts of the body, without blood issuing thence, are a certain mark of possession?

All these questions, to the credit of medical science, were answered in the negative. No one can read them without being struck with the absolute identity of the symptoms, in all essential characteristics, with those which in our day are asserted to be due to spiritual possession, and with those met with in the various forms of hysteria. Cases almost exactly in point have already been cited in this essay.

Nicholas Remigius, judge of the Criminal Court of Lorraine, who in the course of his official career, caused eight hundred women to be burned for sorcery, believed that magic was prevalent far and near around him. This became with him a fixed idea, a veritable madness. He wished to preach a crusade against the sorcerers with whom he believed Europe to be filled. Desperate when he was not believed on his word, that every one was guilty of magic, he ended by declaring himself to be a sorcerer, and on his own confession was burned at the stake.* Can any fact indicate more strongly than this, the overwhelming influence of a strongly rooted belief and the danger of allowing the mind to become possessed with one idea?

Nor have these epidemics been restricted to convents or catholic lands. Protestants of the straitest sects have been visited, and our country has afforded many notable examples, besides possessing the doubtful honor of originating spiritualism in its present form.

The history of witchcraft, as it existed in New England during the latter part of the seventeenth century, is exceedingly instructive to the student of human nature, and of great interest in the present connection. As an illustration of the symptoms exhibited by the so-called "possessed"—the "mediums" of our day—I subjoin the following case, being the "ninth example" adduced by the Rev. Cotton Mather.† It would be difficult to select from all the records of medicine better examples of the blending of hysteria, chorea, and catalepsy. The evidence concerning the diabolical character of the "Quaker's book," "popish books," and the "Prayer-book," is incidentally, though with manifest gusto, thrown in by the narrator for what it is worth.

Four children of John Goodwin, of Boston, remarkable for their piety, honesty, and industry, were in the year 1688 made the subjects of witchcraft. The eldest, a girl about thirteen

* Dogme et Rituel de la Haute Magie Par Elaphas Levi. Paris, 1861, Tome second, p. 290.

† "Magnalia Christi Americana," etc. First American, from the London edition of 1702. Hartford, 1820 vol ii., p. 396.

years old, had a dispute with the laundress about some linen that was missing, whose mother, a "scandalous Irishwoman of the neighborhood," applied some very abusive language to the child. The latter was at once taken with "odd fits, which carried in them something diabolical." Soon afterwards the other children, a girl and two boys, became similarly affected. Sometimes they were deaf, sometimes blind, sometimes dumb, and sometimes all of these. Their tongues would be drawn down their throats, and then pulled out upon their chins to a prodigious length. Their mouths were often forced open to such an extent that their jaws were dislocated, and were then suddenly closed with a snap like that of a spring-lock. The like took place with their shoulders, elbows, wrists, and other joints. They would then lie in a benumbed condition, and be drawn together like those tied neck and heels, and presently be stretched out, and then drawn back enormously. They made piteous outcries that they were cut with knives, and struck with blows, and the plain prints of the wounds were seen upon them.

[This latter is not an uncommon occurrence. I once detected a woman cutting herself with a knife, and thus inflicting wounds which she afterwards declared were given her by a spirit whom she had offended in the flesh.]

At times their necks were rendered so limber that the bones could not be felt, and again they were so stiff that they could not be bent by any degree of force.

The woman who by her spells was supposed to have caused these "possessions," was arrested. Her house was searched, and several images made of rags and stuffed with goat's-hair, were found. These the woman confessed she employed for the purpose of producing the torments in the children, which she did by wetting her finger with saliva and stroking the images. The experiment was made in court, to the entire satisfaction of all concerned. The woman, who was evidently insane, and probably rendered so by the accusations made against her, acknowledged that she was in league with the devil. She was tried, condemned to death, and executed. On the scaffold she declared that others remained who would carry on the work of tormenting the children; and so the calamities of the victims went on. They barked like dogs, purred like cats, at times complained that they were in a red-hot oven, and again that cold water was thrown on them. Then they were roasted on an invisible spit, and would shriek with agony; their heads they said were nailed to the floor, and it was beyond ordinary strength to pull them up. They would be so limber sometimes, that it was judged every bone they had might be bent, and then so stiff that not a joint could be flexed. And so the story goes on through several pages of details. Unseen ropes and chains were put around them, blows were given, and then the narrator continues, in regard to the eldest of the children, who was specially under his observation:—

"A Quaker's book being brought to her, she could quietly read whole pages of it; only the name of God and Christ she still skipped over, being unable to pronounce it, except sometimes stammering a minute or two or more over it. And when we urged her to tell what the word was that she missed, she would say: 'I must not speak it. They say I must not. You know what it is. 'Tis G, and O, and D.' But a book against

Quakerism they would not allow her to meddle with. Such books as it might have been profitable and edifying for her to read, and especially her catechisms, if she did but offer to read a line in them, she would be cast into hideous convulsions, and be tossed about the house like a football. But books of jest being shown her, she could read them well enough, and have cunning descants upon them. Popish books they would not hinder her from reading, but they would from books against popery.

"Divers of these trials were made by many witnesses, but I, considering that there might be a snare in it, put a seasonable stop to this kind of business. Only I could not but be amazed at one thing. A certain prayer-book being brought to her, she not only could read it very well, but also did read a large part of it over, calling it her Bible, and putting a more than ordinary respect upon it. If she were going into her tortures, at the tender of this book, she would recover herself to read it."

Then she rode invisible horses, and continued other pranks, till at last "one particular minister" (who seems to have been very negligent heretofore), "taking a peculiar compassion on the family, set himself to serve them in the methods prescribed by our Lord Jesus Christ. Accordingly, the Lord being besought thrice in three days of prayer, with fasting, on this occasion, the family then saw their deliverance perfected."

In the tenth example it is stated that one Winlock Curtis, a sailor, "was violently and suddenly seized in an unaccountable manner, and furiously thrown down upon the deck, where he lay wallowing in a great agony, and foamed at the mouth, and grew black in the face, and was near strangled with a great lump rising in his neck nigh his throat, like that which bewitched or possessed people used to be attended withal." Winlock Curtis clearly had an epileptic fit, and the lump spoken of was the well-known globus hystericus, which few of my nervous readers have failed to experience at some time or other of their lives.

Finally, the epidemic spread with such rapidity, and so many accused themselves of converse with the devil, that the common-sense of the people put a stop to further executions. In the language of Mather, "Experience showed that the more there were apprehended the more were still afflicted by Satan, and the number of confessions increasing did but increase the number of the accused; and the executing of some made way for the apprehending of others. For still the afflicted complained of being tormented by new objects, as the former were removed. So that those that were concerned grew amazed at the number and quality of the persons accused, and feared that Satan by his wiles had enwrapped innocent persons under the imputation of that crime; and at last it was evidently seen that there must be a stop put, or the generation of the children of God would fall under that condemnation. Henceforth, therefore, the juries generally acquitted such as were tried, fearing they had gone too far before, and Sir William Phips, the governor, reprieved all that were condemned, even the confessors as well as others."

The epidemic, being thus let alone, died a natural death, as would likewise be the case with the spiritualism of the present day with similar treatment.

The vagaries of the shakers and jumpers of our own country, and of the whirling dervishes and other sects of the old world, and the contortions, trances, and beatifications of camp-meetings and revivals, may also receive a portion of our attention.

McNemar,* who was an eye witness of what he describes, but whose book has almost passed out of sight, says of the Kentucky revival :—

"At first appearance these meetings exhibited nothing to the spectator but a scene of confusion, that could scarcely be put into any language. They were generally opened with a sermon, near the close of which there would be an unusual outcry, even bursting out into loud ejaculations of prayer, etc.

"The rolling exercise consisted in being cast down in a violent manner, doubled with the head and feet together, or stretched in a prostrate manner, turning swiftly over like a dog. Nothing in nature could better represent the jerks than for one to goad another alternately on every side with a red-hot iron. The exercise commonly began in the head, which would fly backwards and forwards and from side to side with a quick jolt, which the person would naturally labor to suppress, but in vain. He must necessarily go on as he was stimulated, whether with a violent dash on the ground and bounce from place to place like a foot-ball, hopping round with head, limbs

* The Kentucky Revival; or, A Short History of the Late Extraordinary Outpouring of the Spirit of God in the Western States of America, agreeable to Scripture Promises and Prophecies concerning the Latter Day. With a brief account of the entrance and progress of what the world calls Shakerism among the subjects of the late revival in Ohio and Kentucky. Presented to the True Zion Traveller as a Memorial of the Wilderness Journey. Cincinnati. 1807.

and trunk twitching and jolting in every direction, as if they must inevitably fly asunder."

Lorenzo Dow, in his *Journal*, states that at one of the meetings at which he preached, at Knoxville, Tennessee, in 1805, a hundred and fifty persons, among them several quakers, were affected with the "jerks." "I have seen," he says, "all denominations of religion exercised by the jerks, gentleman and lady, black and white, young and old, without exception. I passed a meeting-house where I observed the undergrowth had been cut down for camp-meetings, and from fifty to a hundred saplings were left for the people who were jerked to hold by. I observed where they had held on, they had kicked up the earth as a horse stamping flies."

Another account of the Kentucky revival is that of Mr. Geo. A. Baxter,* a man of whom the Rev. Archibald Alexander, President of Hampden Sidney College in Virginia, says, "I never knew a man in whose judgment in a matter of this kind I could more confidently rely."

The account states that the people were accustomed to assemble on sacramental occasions to the number of from eight to twelve thousand, and to continue on the ground in devotional exercises for several days and nights. They were addressed by several ministers, and presently some of the audience began to fall down, which at first created some disorder, but soon this fall became so general and frequent that it excited no disturbance. At Cane-Ridge sacrament, it was

* Quoted by Dr. Brigham from the *Connecticut Evangelical Magazine*, Vol. II., in Observations on the Influence of Religion upon the Health. Boston, 1855, p. 229.

generally supposed that not less than one thousand persons fell prostrate to the ground, and among them many infidels. At one sacrament at which Mr. Baxter attended, the number that fell was thought to be over three thousand. It was common to see the fallers shed tears plentifully for about an hour. Then they were seized with a general tremor, and sometimes they uttered, at the moment of falling, piercing shrieks. Sometimes they could not sit up or speak, the pulse became weak and the breathing very slow. At others, all signs of life left them, for an hour or more. In many cases the falling was very sudden; some would go down as if struck by lightning. Many infidels and other vicious characters were arrested in this way, and sometimes at the very moment in which they were uttering their blasphemies against the work.

On one occasion he says:—"The people, as usual, met on Friday, but they were all languid, and the exercises went on heavily. On Saturday and Sunday morning it was no better. At length the communion service commenced, and everything was still lifeless. The minister of the place was speaking at one of the tables without any unusual liberty. All at once there were several shrieks from different parts of the assembly. Persons fell instantly in every direction. The feelings of the hearers were suddenly relieved, and the work went on with extraordinary power from that time to the conclusion of the solemnity."

And all this was called "The outpouring of the Holy Spirit!"

Some ministers were then, as now, more potent to convert than others. Thus, one of the most gifted in this respect, at least in his own estimation, was the Rev. Mr. Foote,* who says, "Most ministers, I suppose, do not expect to convert a hundred souls in all their lives; but though I am a poor creature, I should not think I did anything unless I converted two thousand or two thousand five hundred a year."

In England, like performances resulted from the ministrations of Mr. Wesley, and are thus described in his Journal:

"Sunday, May 20, being with Mr. B—ll, at Everton, I was much fatigued and did not rise, but Mrs. B—— did, and observed many fainting and crying out, while Mr. Berridge was preaching; afterwards, at church, I heard many cry out, especially children, whose agonies were amazing; one of the oldest, a girl of ten or twelve years old, was full in my view, in violent contortions of body, and weeping aloud, I think, incessantly during the whole service; and several much younger children were in Mr. B—ll's full view, agonizing as they did. The church was equally crowded in the afternoon, the windows being filled within and without, and even the outside of the pulpit to the very top, so that Mr. B—— seemed almost stifled with their breath; yet feeble and sickly as he is, he was continually strengthened, and his voice, for the most part, distinguishable in the midst of all the outcries. I believe there were present three times more men than women, a greater part of whom came from afar; thirty of them having set out at two in the morning, from a place thirteen miles off. The text was: '*Having a fear of godliness but denying the power thereof.*' When the power of religion began to be spoken of, the pres-

* "Account of the Seven Protracted Meetings in Berkshire Co., Mass." By the Rev. D. D. Field, of Stockbridge. *Boston Recorder*, April 3, 1835, cited by Brigham, op. cit., p. 242.

ence of God really filled the place; and while poor sinners felt the sentence of death in their souls, what sounds of distress did I hear! The greatest number of those who cried or fell, were men; but some women and several children felt the power of the same almighty spirit, and seemed just sinking into hell. This occasioned a mixture of various sounds; some shrieking, some roaring aloud. The most general was a loud breathing like that of people half strangled and gasping for life; and, indeed, almost all the cries were like those of human creatures dying in bitter anguish. Great numbers wept without any noise; others fell down as dead; some sinking in silence; some with extreme noise and violent agitation. I stood on the pew seat, as did a young man on the opposite pew, an able-bodied, fresh, healthy countryman; but in a moment, while he seemed to think of nothing less, down he dropped with a violence inconceivable. The adjoining pew seemed to shake with his fall. I heard afterwards the stamping of his feet; ready to break the boards as he lay in strong convulsions at the bottom of the pew. Among several that were struck down in the next pew, was a girl who was as violently seized as he. When he fell, Mr. B—ll and I felt our souls thrilled with a momentary dread; as when one man is killed with a cannon-ball another often feels the wind of it.

"Among the children who felt the arrows of the Almighty, I saw a sturdy boy about eight years old, who roared above his fellows, and seemed, in his agony, to struggle with the strength of a grown man. His face was red as scarlet, and almost all on whom God laid his hand, turned either very red or almost black. When I returned after a little walk to Mr. Berridge's house, I found it full of people. He was fatigued, but said he would nevertheless give them a word of exhortation. I stayed in the next room and saw the girl whom I had observed so peculiarly distressed in the church, lying on the floor as one dead, but without any ghastliness in her face. In a few minutes we were informed of a woman filled with peace and joy, who was crying out just before. She had come thirteen miles, and is the same person who dreamed Mr. B—— would come to her village on that very day whereon he did come, though without either knowing the place or the way to it. She was convinced at that time. Just as we heard of her deliverance, the girl on the floor began to stir. She was then set on a chair; and after sighing awhile, suddenly rose up rejoicing in God. Her face was covered with the most beautiful smile I ever saw. She frequently fell on her knees but was generally running to and fro, speaking these and the like words: 'Oh, what can Jesus do for lost sinners? He has forgiven all my sins! I am in heaven! I am in heaven! Oh, how he loves *me!* And how I love him!' Meantime, I saw a thin, pale girl, weeping with sorrow for herself and joy for her companion. Quickly the smiles of heaven came likewise on her, and her praises joined with those of the other. I also then laughed with extreme joy, so did Mr. B—ll (who said it was more than he could well bear). So did all who knew the Lord, and some of those who were waiting for salvation, till the cries of those who were struck with the arrows of conviction, were almost lost in the sounds of joy. * * * *

"Immediately after a stranger, well dressed, who stood facing me, fell backward to the wall; then forward on his knees, wringing his hands and roaring like a bull. His face at first turned quite red and then almost black. He rose and ran against the wall, till Mr. Keeling and another held him. He screamed out, 'Oh, what shall I do, what shall I do? Oh, for one drop of the blood of Christ!' As he spoke, God set his soul at liberty; he knew his sins were blotted out; and the raptures he was in seemed too great for human nature to bear. He had come forty miles to hear Mr. B——, and was to leave the next morning; which he did with a glad heart, telling all who came in his way, what God had done for his soul. * * *

"And now did I see such a sight as I do not expect again on this side eternity. The faces of the three justified children, and I think of all the believers present, did really shine; and such a beauty, such a look of extreme happiness and at the same time of divine love and simplicity, did I never see in human faces till now. The newly justified eagerly embraced one another, weeping on each other's necks for joy. Then they saluted all of their own sex and besought men and women to help them in praising God."

On the 24th, Mr. Wesley went to hear Mr. Hicks preach at Wrestlingworth, and thus describes what ensued:

"While he was preaching, fifteen or sixteen persons felt the arrows of the Lord and dropped down. A few of these cried out with the utmost violence, and little intermission for some hours, while the rest made no great noise but continued struggling as in the pangs of death. I observed besides them, one little girl deeply convinced, and a boy nine or ten years old, both of them, and several others, when carried into the parsonage house, either lay as dead or struggled with all their might, but in a short time their cries increased beyond measure, so that the loudest singing could scarcely be heard. Some at last called on me to pray, which I did, and for a time all were calm; but the storm soon began again."

This is not all. There is a great deal more to the same effect, and were it not that there is such a condition as hysteria, we should be disposed to take the other alternative of demoniacal possession, as an explanation of the frightful orgies, which under the blasphemous designation of the "outpouring of the spirit of God," excelled in hideousness the frenzies of the demonolaters of the East.

Hysteria from any other cause is marked by exactly such phenomena—the emotional disturbance, the falling, the loss of consciousness, the spasms, convulsions, coma, are all so many symptoms which physicians see every day arise from very different factors than the "spirit of God." The well-known force of contagion by example, has no more marked exponent than hysteria affords, and hence, when one began to sob, and to be convulsed, to cry out in agony and to fall in a coma, the spark was set to the train, and the others with pent-up emotions, were ready to do likewise.

But the relations of hysteria to religion have never been more distinctly shown than in the fact that women under its influence, have been able to gather numerous followers and actually to originate new religious faiths, of such preposterous tenets and practices, as to inevitably lead to the conclusion that the adherents are either fools or knaves.

Take for instance, the shakers. This sect professes to believe that Christ made his second appearance on earth in the person of one Ann Lee, an Englishwoman, daughter of James Lee, a blacksmith of Manchester, England. This woman was employed in a hat manufactory, was married when very young, and had four or five children all of whom died in infancy. At a very early period of her life, Ann Lee began to feel the "awful sinfulness of sin and the depth of man's fall." Although she could neither read nor write, she managed to pick up from others a little smattering of the Bible, and evinced a great interest in the Apocrypha, as was natural she should, under the peculiar circumstances of her career. She always said the Apocrypha was the cream of the Bible.

Night and day she labored to discover the root of all evil, and being convinced beyond a doubt where it lay, she opened a flaming testimony against it, which called down upon her head showers of persecutions, too cruel for long endurance. But many adopted her views and she was called "mother," as the head of the band of followers she had gathered around her.

By continual fasting and prayer, much agony of soul, incessant cries, tears and entreaties by day and by night, she wasted away, till becoming helpless, her followers were under the necessity of taking her in their arms as an infant. It is said she was fed with pap from a spoon, the greater portion of the time during which she was travailing in the "New Birth." She travailed nine years in this way, and then she announced that she was born again "completely redeemed from all the propensities of a fallen nature, in July, 1790." She then separated from her husband and was duly regarded as the second Christ—the Redeemer of the world.

Like all new religions, this met with violent persecution—not enough to crush it, just enough to feed it. In every place in England in which Mother Ann undertook to worship God by dancing on Sunday and preaching against the institution of marriage, persecution was excited; but she bore up against it and her followers increased.

As in the case of other originators of religious dogmas, which do not admit of proof, Mother Ann began to work miracles for the confusion of the unbelievers, and the strengthening of the convictions of the faithful.

Thus we are told she was dragged before the magistrates, for no other offence than worshipping God in the way laid down by herself, and was condemned to a cold, dark prison, with a small allowance of bread and water; yet she lived, to the great astonishment and confusion of her enemies. After being confined in this dark prison, in delicate health, and with insufficient food, the doors were thrown open, and thousands of spectators in breathless anxiety awaited the egress of an emaciated and subdued woman, supported by one of her followers; but to their great astonishment Mother Ann came forth in unsurpassed beauty, with an air of dignified buoyancy, a halo of glory around her head, singing a song of paradise given her by an angel who attended her in the prison, and who had fed her with food sent by the Eternal Mother. For the Shakers worship a quadruple God, consisting of the Eternal Father, the Eternal Mother, the Son and Holy Ghost, corresponding to Power, Mother Ann, Jesus Christ and Wisdom.

This miraculous event so incensed the people that she was taken, with her followers, to a valley a short distance from

Manchester. The mob collected on a hill near by, and commenced a furious attack on them with stones and other missiles. These projectiles flew with tremendous velocity till within a few inches of their object, and then fell harmless to the ground. Mother Ann saw a circle of power of God around about them like a high wall.

Then they determined to leave a country where they met with so little appreciation, and so set sail for America. On the voyage Mother Ann stilled a raging tempest, and kept the sea calm till they landed. She died in a few years, and took her place in heaven, to be worshipped as a member of the Godhead.*

The religious ceremonial of these degraded creatures has no one redeeming feature about it. The demonolatrous worship of the Hindoos has an object—the propitiation of a powerful being—but the shaker ritual is abjectly degrading to human nature, without even the excuse of adoration.

There are many among them who profess to see God, Christ and Mother Ann. They are taken to the spiritual world and introduced to good spirits, where they often sit at table with the Godhead. At their meetings, some one called the visionist directs the proceedings. Standing at the head of the room, this person, who professes to see God, Christ or Mother Ann, and to be in communion with them, gives his orders to the assembled people. He calls on one to step forth and shake. The victim comes forward, drops his or her hands to the side,

* This account, as well as what follows, is quoted in an abridged form from "Extract from an Unpublished Manuscript on Shaker History; by an Eye Witness." Boston, 1850.

and begins shaking the whole body and stamping with the feet, while the visionist calls out at the top of his voice "Shake! Shake! Shake! There is a great spirit on you, shake him off! shake him off! Christ says, shake him off!" Another then takes up the cry: "Down! down! come down! Christ says, come down! Low! low! low!" At which every person in the room bends and bows like willows in a high wind. Sometimes one of the gifted, will see the devil come into the meeting, and, like a faithful sentinel, gives the alarm, when every true believer opens the battery at once by drawing the right arm nearly to the chin, placing the arm in the position as if to shoot, and then straightening the body out with a jerk and a stamp of the foot, accompanied by a quick bursting yelp in imitation of a gun, all being the work of a moment. "There," says the visionist, "see him dart; he has gone down towards the chimney; shoot him! shoot him! kill him!" and a rush is made for spiritual weapons, given by the visionist from the spiritual armory.

Sometimes Christ or Mother Ann enters the meeting-room, bearing such presents as the band wants. These presents are "spiritual," and are handed round by Christ to the faithful, who receive them as though they were real gifts. To one golden potatoes are given; to another, oranges; to others, cake, puddings, jellies, etc., with various other things not known to this world.

Mother Ann has a splendid vineyard; the walks are of pure gold, with angels walking around among the vines. There are ten thousand kinds of grapes. Mother Ann superintends her own wine press, and often brings wine ("spiritual" again) as a present. The visionist pretends to take a waiter filled with wine-glasses ; every body must have faith, and take one as it is handed to them. Those who have little or no faith are told by the visionist whether they have taken theirs. Then they all raise their hands to their lips as in the act of drinking, and presently they begin to reel and stagger around the room as though actually drunk. Indeed, they act in all respects as drunken persons, stamping, shaking, vomiting, etc., till finally, exhausted, they gradually sink away till all is silent. Then, standing in a circle, they throw their handkerchiefs over their shoulders, raise their hands to their heads, and make six solemn bows, saying with each, "I kindly thank Mother for this beautiful gift."

Often some one will feel a "laughing gift," and will begin with—he, he, he ; ha, ha, ha ; ho, ho, ho. Another takes it up, and soon all in the room are engaged in boisterous laughter. Once under full "laughing gift," they will hold on to their sides and reel in their chairs till they become exhausted. This gift ends in a song:

Ho, ho, ho ; he, he, he ;
O, what a pretty little path I see :
Pretty path, pretty play,
Pretty little angels,
Hay, hay, hay.

The first and last lines are sung with a loud laugh.

A gift sometimes called the "mortification gift" enters the room. One might suppose it came direct from the barn-yard, as the inspired begin slapping their hands against their sides and crowing in imitation of a chicken-cock. Some will cackle, others imitate the turkey, duck, hen, goose, or guinea-fowl.

Sometimes young men and women are exercised by what they call the "jerks," for two weeks at a time, during the whole of which period the head is kept in continual motion by quick, convulsive motions of the shoulders and neck. The author of the little book from which these particulars are quoted says she once saw a young woman whose face was frightfully swollen, her eyes dilated and bloodshot, and who had been exercised by the "jerks" for three weeks. Directly after the "jerks" she began to talk in unknown tongues, and continued at short intervals for three or four days; then she stopped suddenly, and remained entirely mute for two weeks, no possible persuasion being sufficient to make her say even yes or no. This experience is called the "dumb devils."

"At one time," she writes, "while in a mission meeting, the visionist said 'Vicalun' was present. I was told that 'Vicalun' was the angel of repentance, and he had come to visit me, if I would 'own the gift.' I informed the visionist that I felt honored by the notice.

"They then sang a very solemn song in 'unknown tongues' and English, called 'Vicalun's Prayer,' reading thus:—

'Hark! hark! my holy, holy,
Vicalun seelen sor,
I have come to mourn
And weep with you
In low humiliation;
Pray to the silun sool,
Whose hand can stay the billows,
And san si rulun sool.'

"I cannot do justice to these songs by writing them. The spiritual gifts are never set to music. They have some excellent songs, however, and very difficult to execute correctly

The song just quoted has a variety of changes, accompanied by the following motions: At the first line the head is inclined forward, with the forefinger pointing to the right ear, as in the act of listening. At the third line the hands are brought forward with an earnest beckoning motion. At the fourth line the hands are carried to the eyes as in the act of weeping, the body gradually bending till it sinks on the knees and the face touches the floor at the close of the fifth line. At the commencement of the sixth line both hands are brought up to the side of the head as in prayer; at the seventh the right hand is thrown convulsively upward; at the word 'Vicalun' both hands are extended wide. At the last line, and at the last word, they are clasped over the heart. The last four lines are repeated twice. Appropriate motions accompany all songs sung by them."

Now, can any person not utterly lost to all sense of the dignity of the human species think of these things without doubting the sanity of those who practise them? In what essential respect do these acts differ from those of the demonolaters, as described by Caldwell? * A devil has been angered, and must be propitiated.

"Beat the tom-tom louder. Let the fattest sheep be offered as a propitiation! Let the horns blaze out as the priest rolls about in the giddy dance, and gashes himself in his frenzy. More fire! Quicker music! Wilder bounds from the devil-dancers! Shrieks and laughter, and sobs, and frantic shouts! And over the long, lone valley, and up the bouldered mountain-side, under the wan moon, thrills out loud and savage and

* "Demonolatry, Devil-Dancing, and Demoniacal Possession." *The Contemporary Review*, Feb., 1876.

shrill, the wild, tremulous wailing of women and yells of maddened men. 'Ha, ha! I am God! God! The God is in me, and shrieks! Come, hasten, tell me all! I will solace you, cure you! God is in me, and I am God! Hack and slaughter! The blood of the sacrifice is sweet! Another fowl! Another goat! Quick, I am athirst for blood! Obey your God!' Such are the words which hoarsely burst from the frothing lips of the devil-dancer, as he bounds and leaps and gyrates, with short, sharp cries, and red eyes almost starting from their sockets."

Mr. Caldwell appears to believe that the devil-dancers are in reality, as they believe, possessed by demons. What would he say if present at some such shaker gatherings as have been described? He and others may believe in possession, but those who know how low the majesty of the human mind can fall, and what strange and degraded acts, hysteria and hysteroid affections lead their subjects to commit, will see only in spiritualism, shakerism, camp-meetings, devil-dancing, and their congeners, fresh reasons to doubt the existence of any very broad line of demarkation between man and the rest of the animal kingdom.

Mr. Wesley, had he been present at a shaker meeting, would doubtless have seen little of the "outpouring of the spirit of God" in their acts. He would probably have regarded the performers as possessed by evil spirits and as mocking the God they pretended to please. But "heterodoxy is your doxy, orthodoxy is my doxy," the world over. This is what the shakers think of him.

"After singing this prayer, the young prophet rose from his seat and approached me saying, "Will you hear what the spirit has to say to you?' I answered, yes. He then returned to his seat and commenced bowing his head as is the custom in the opening of a 'gift,' and said, 'O, look there and see that great spirit! He has got a large rope in his hand and it is tied around your waist; and O look! there is another on the other side, he has got a rope around your waist. There! see him pull you.' I asked him who these spirits were. 'Why,' said he, 'Christ says, the one on your left side is John Wesley, and the other on your right side is John Murray. First you incline to the one and then to the other. But oh look, there is an awful spirit! He has got a great iron chain around both these men. O mother, do tell us who that awful spirit is!' After a moment's pause, he exclaimed, 'Why it is the devil! so you see, let you go to either of these men, you will go to the devil, for he has them both.' I asked him why I did not go if Murray, Wesley and the Devil had united their forces to draw me with cable ropes and iron chains? The young man sat a moment and then said, 'Oh, I see it all now; there is a beautiful spirit all light and glory, right behind you. Dear, good spirit, do tell me what you are, so very glorious? Why now I know, it is our blessed mother, and she has got a splendid gold chain around your waist, holding your arm, so you had better let methodism and universalism alone, and cheat the devil by being a good child of mother's kingdom.'"

Again, there is the remarkable example of Joanna Southcott, who announcing that she had conceived by supernatural agency and was about to give birth to a second Christ, or rather that Christ was to be born again through her, obtained many followers who anxiously expected the promised advent. She called herself the woman spoken of in the Revelation of St. John, as the "Bride, the Lamb's Wife clothed with the sun," as she said,* "by types, shadows, dreams and visions, I have been led on from 1792 to the present day."

Day and night she had hallucinations or visions, as she called them, which she accepted as realities, and which formed the basis of her prophecies and system of religion. Meetings were held to inquire into the truth of her pretensions, and at once a court was organized and a trial instituted. The result was that she was accepted for all she claimed to be, as the document was published, worded as follows:

"We, whose names are hereunto subscribed, being invited by divine command for seven days to the examination of Joanna Southcote, do individually and voluntarily avow by our separate signatures, our firm belief that her prophecies and other spiritual communications, emanate wholly and entirely from the Spirit of the living Lord."

And among the names subscribed to this precious instrument of human folly, are those of several of the clergy!

She was subject to paroxsyms of weeping, to trances and convulsions of a hysterical character. She often saw and conversed with the devil, and his satanic majesty did not hesitate to abuse and threaten her in language scarce fit for polite ears. "Thou infamous ——," said Satan, enraged at the opposition he met with, "thou hast been flattering God that He may stand thy friend! Such low cunning I despise! Thou scheming wretch,

* "The Strange Effects of Faith with Remarkable Prophecies (made in 1792, etc.) of Things which are to come; also, Some Account of My Life." Printed for the author. Exeter, 1801. p. 16.

stop thy —— eternal tongue! God has done something to choose a —— of a woman that will argue down the devil and scarce give him room to speak." *

On other occasions she was visited by Christ. It is painful to be obliged to refer to such events, but it must be remembered that this woman was sincere, actually believing in the reality of all she imagined she saw, and thousands of others drinking in as truth, every word that fell from her lips or pen.

"Who," says the author from whom I have just quoted, "can peruse the account of the following vision, for example, related by Miss Townley in the pamphlet entitled 'Letters and Communications of Joanna Southcott,' and not be staggered at the disclosure of such scenes? Monday evening, July 2d, 1804, it seems that Joanna tried to compose herself after a hard contest with the devil, when " at last she fell asleep, and whether awake or asleep," continues Miss Townley, "she does not know, but she remembers she was quite awake when she felt the hand of the Lord upon her, but in that heavenly and beautiful manner, that she felt joy unspeakable and full of glory. She felt herself lying as it were, in heaven, in the hands of the Lord, and was afraid to move fearing she should remove his heavenly hand, which she felt as perfect as ever woman felt the hand of her husband." Here the "Lamb's Wife" herself, takes up the tale. 'In this happy manner,' affirms

* Memoirs of the Life and Mission of Joanna Southcott, interspersed with authentic anecdotes and elucidated by interesting documents; including the Progress of her Pregnancy, detailed by Herself, together with the opinions of Drs. Reece and Sims, to which is added a Sketch of the Rev. W. Tozer, M.J.S., embellished with a likeness of the Prophetess. London, 1814, p. 15.

Joanna, 'I fell asleep, and in my sleep I was surprised with seeing a most beautiful and heavenly figure that arose from the bed between Townley and me. He arose and turned himself backwards towards the foot of the bed, and his head almost reached the tester of the bed, but his face was towards me, which appeared with beauty and majesty, but pale as death. His hair was a flaxen color, all in disorder around his face. His face was covered with strong perspiration and his locks were wet like the dew of night, as though they had been taken out of a river. The collar of his shirt appeared unbuttoned, and the skin of his bosom appeared white as the driven snow. Such was the beauty of the heavenly figure that appeared before me in a disordered state; but the robe he had on was like a surplice down to his knees. He put out one of his legs to me, that was perfectly like mine, no larger, but with purple spots at the top, as mine are with beating myself, which Townley, Underwood, and Taylor, are witnesses of. Methought in my dream, he got himself into that perspiration by being pressed to sleep between Townley and me. I said to him, 'are you my dear dying Saviour that is come to destroy all the works of the devil?' He answered, 'Yes.' I thought I called Underwood and waked Townley, to look at him, which they did with wonder and amaze."

Such sexual orgasms were frequently misinterpreted by the mystical women of the middle ages, into acts of intercourse with angels and members of the Godhead, so that Joanna's experience was not isolated.

Then, when in her sixty-fifth year, she gave out that her pregnancy had at last occurred, and that Christ would be born again of her, several medical men examined her and certified that she was actually pregnant. But a Dr. Sims took another view of the case, and gave his views at length, for arriving at a contrary opinion.

Nevertheless, the faithful continued to believe. A crib of satin wood, mounted in gold, was provided for the heavenly infant. This was called "the manger." Bed-clothing of the finest linen, lace, satin and silk, embroidered with doves and trimmed with gold lace, was supplied, and the bed was of eider-down. The whole cost upwards of two hundred pounds.

The time arrived, her adherents waited patiently, but there was no birth. Excuses were made, and the number of her followers scarcely diminished during her lifetime.

It is hardly credible that human folly can reach to such extremes, as it is shown to have attained in the development of Shakerism and the delusions of Joanna Southcote. We shall, however, see that there are still lower depths. That Spiritualism, therefore, should have its adherents, need excite no surprise. A little inquiry into the operations of the human mind, as they relate to matters of faith, is sufficient to reveal to us the fact that the extent of human credulity is illimitable, and that nothing can be asserted so absurd, so degrading, so blasphemous, so impossible, that there will not be found men and women with minds badly enough organized, to accept it as an article of belief.

In a recent work,* which certainly may be regarded as good

* Modern American Spiritualism; a Twenty Years Record of the Communion between Earth and Heaven. By Emma Hardinge. Second Edition. New York, 1870, p. 159.

spiritualistic authority, there is an account of a medium who was by turns under the influence of a good spirit called, 'Katy,' and of a bad one whom she asserted to be a 'sailor boy.' This latter, took great delight in swearing through her and in uttering such profane language as he had been accustomed to on earth. Many manifestations of the power of these spirits were given:

"About 1846, a most singular and distressing phase of these phenomena was superadded to the rest, under what claimed to be the influence of the profane sailor. The girl's limbs in several directions, would be thrown out of joint and that with apparent ease, in a moment and without pain. To replace them seemed to be either beyond the power or the will of her invisible tormentor, and Dr. Larkin, (a weak minded man, whose servant she was) though an experienced surgeon, was often obliged to call in the aid of his professional brethren, and his or their strong assistants.

"On one occasion the knees and wrists of the girl were thrown out of joint, twice in a single day. Those painful feats were always accompanied by loud laughter, hoarse and profane jokes, and expressions of exultant delight, purporting to come from the sailor, while the girl herself seemed wholly unconscious of the danger of her awkward situation. The preternatural feats of agility and strength exhibited on these occasions could scarcely be credited, and the frightfully unnatural contortions of the limbs with which she became tied up into knots and coils, baffle all physiological explanation or attempts at description.

This last statement arises from Mrs. Hardinge's ignorance of the capacities of hysteria. Can any body familiar with its vagaries doubt for an instant that this girl was suffering from it, and that her condition was aggravated by the notoriety which she gained by her performances? In what respect do these so-called spiritualistic exhibitors differ from those which have been cited, and, except in being less strongly marked, from those to which attention will be asked in the following chapter.

But though we can deplore the ignorance of those who believed this girl to be possessed by two spirits, what are we to think of the lamentable darkness in which certain of her neighbours seemed to have lived. Mrs. Hardinge* makes the statement that the Rev. Horace James, one of the ministers of Wrentham in the year 1849, and an unceasing slanderer and persecutor of Dr. Larkin, summoned three magistrates, who, together with a few persons of the place, inimical to the manifestations, constituted a judicial court, before which Dr. Larkin was cited to appear, and on authority of which the unfortunate sick girl was dragged from her bed and arrested on the charge of "necromancy!"

In this notable case the Rev. Horace James, according to Mrs. Hardinge, appeared as complainant, chief witness, and even judge.

"If," says Mrs. Hardinge, "the details of this unheard of court of justice should seem to draw too largely on the credulity of nineteenth century readers, if it seems impossible to believe that in 1849 a poor sick girl could be dragged from her bed on the charge of 'necromancy,' and a respectable physician hauled before a court of his own neighbors on a charge of sorcery, let

* Op. cit., p. 162.

the sequel speak for itself. Mary Jane was convicted on this charge and and actually sentenced to sixty days' confinement in Dedham jail: witness the Dedham jail records in the State of Massachusetts."

This seems almost incredible, but the account is circumstantial, and has never, to my knowledge, been denied.

From the same volume* the following account is taken:—

"Four badly-educated girls, of ages ranging from fifteen to twenty, having gathered together at a friend's house to have a time with the spirits, or, in other words, to trifle with spiritual manifestations, seated themselves around a table, and after asking all manner of foolish questions, requested the spirits to lay hold of them.

"The spirits at once complied, seized them, treated them in the roughest manner, and, shaking them, caused them to use the most violent actions and outrageous language, etc. In this strait one of the dignitaries of the mother church was sent for in haste to 'expel the obsessing demons.' After the priest had arrived at the scene of disorder, he put on his robes, got ready the holy water, and approached the possessed girls in the due formulæ proper to such occasions. After many sallies with the holy fluid, and a vast number of incantations, none of which produced the slightest effect, the mediums at length charged upon him with such irresistible power and such capacity of finger-nails, that the worthy *padre* fled precipitately, leaving the field in possession of the 'demons' and the spectators who had gathered together to witness the 'exorcism.' The girls still continued to be used roughly, by the discordant spirits they

* Op. cit., p. 271.

had invoked, until the arrival of some of their spiritualistic friends, by whose judicious passes and gentle remonstrances with the spirits, they were instantly relieved."

That these " silly, badly-educated girls " were simply hysterical, no one with even a superficial acquaintance with the normal condition of the nervous system, and the aberrations to which it may be subjected, can entertain the slightest doubt. It is from just such persons as these that the best mediums are obtained. That such phenomena as they and the girl whose case was previously quoted, exhibited are regarded as spiritualistic, is sufficient of itself to throw discredit on all the other alleged manifestations of the spirits." "*Falsum in uno, falsum in omnibus.*"

At most of the spiritualistic meetings which the writer has attended there have been hysterical phenomena manifested by some of the men and women participating in the exercises. At a recent public exhibition of the kind he predicted, from their personal appearance, with perfect accuracy who of those assisting would be thus affected. The symptoms of disordered nervous action which the audience was invited to consider proofs of spiritual agency consisted of incoherent utterances and convulsive movements of the head, arms, and legs. In one case these symptoms became permanent for several months; a well-developed case of chorea, or St. Vitus's dance was thus established. The patient finally came under the writer's care, and was only cured by the persistent administration of iron and strychnine—medicines which, with good food and fresh air, appear to possess more exorcising power than the formulæ of the good priest mentioned by Mrs. Hardinge.

In hysteria, hallucinations of the several senses are very common. Attention has already been directed to the fact that they may be produced by an excessive amount of blood circulating through the brain. Hysteria is always accompanied by an anæmic condition of the brain, and hence we have an illustration of the well-known fact that opposite pathological states may give rise to similar sets of symptoms. It frequently happens that, just before death from exhausting diseases, the brain, enfeebled with the other organs of the body, is deceived by hallucinations of sight and hearing.

The records of spiritualism abound with instances of spirits being seen by the faithful, and many of the cases are to be referred to the existence of hysteria.* From among numerous similar examples which have come under the professional care or observation of the writer, the following are adduced :—

A young lady gave very decided evidence of suffering from mental aberration. She had imbibed the delusion that she had a "double," whom she saw almost constantly, and with whom she conversed whenever she pleased. At first she had been very much frightened, but gradually had become accustomed to her imaginary companion, and was lonesome and uncomfortable without her. There was no other well-marked delusion, though some of her absurd fancies partook more or less of that character. Headache was almost an inseparable symptom, as was likewise pain in the back, nausea, and constipation. Her menstrual function was deranged, and her whole aspect was that of a

* For a very philosophical account of hallucinations due to slight cerebral disturbance, the reader is referred to "An Essay toward a Theory of Apparitions," by John Ferriar, M.D. London, 1813.

person whose physical powers were below par. Strychnia, iron, and whiskey, and a full, nutritious diet, were not long in banishing her delusional visitor, and in otherwise restoring her health.

A married lady consulted the writer for advice regarding hallucinations of sight and hearing, with which she had suffered for several months. It was only necessary for her to think of some particular person, living or dead, when she immediately saw the image of the person thought of, who spoke to her, laughed, wept, walked about the room, or did whatever other thing she imagined. In fact, to such an extent had her proclivity reached, that it was often impossible for her to avoid thinking of persons, and immediately having their figures brought to her perception.

At first she religiously believed in the reality of her visions, and that she really saw the spirits of the various individuals of whom she happened to think. But, as the hallucinations became more common, she lost her faith, and ascribed them to their true cause—disease. Upon examination, I found that she was preëminently of an hysterical type of organization, and was then laboring under other symptoms of its presence, besides the hallucinations. Thus she had hysterical paralysis of motion and sensation in the right leg, to such an extent that she could neither move it, nor feel a pin thrust through the skin ; there was occasional loss of voice and of the power of speech, and tonic contractions of various muscles, especially of those of the fingers and toes. Her pulse was small and weak, her bowels obstinately constipated, her appetite capricious, and her complexion pale. Not the least of her afflictions was an almost perpetual headache. Under a suitable hygienic and medicinal treatment, this lady entirely recovered.

A young lady, whom I saw at Bridgeport, Connecticut, in consultation with my friends Drs. Hubbard and Ohnesorg, had hallucinations of sight, in conjunction with other symptoms of the hysterical condition.

Another, whom I visited in consultation with my friend Dr. Blakeman, of this city, constantly saw a man, armed with a gun, whom she called Peter, and with whom she carried on a conversation. She described him in detail, and tried to make others see him.

Another young lady, in regard to whom I was not long since consulted, was subject to fallings like those described by Mr. Wesley, convulsions and trances, during which she had visions of various kinds, as the result of emotional disturbance of even the slightest description. Upon one occasion she lay in a trance for seventeen hours, because a dress which had been made for her was not trimmed exactly to her liking; and on another had a violent epileptiform convulsion, during which she foamed at the mouth, because a novel she was reading turned out differently from her expectations.

Occasionally persons have the power of voluntarily producing hallucinations of various kinds—a practice fraught with danger, for the time comes, sooner or later, in which they cannot get rid of their false perceptions. Goethe states that he had the power of giving form to the images passing before his mind, and on one occasion saw his own figure approaching him. Abercrombie* refers to the case of a gentleman who had all

* Inquiries concerning the Intellectual Powers, and the Investigation of Truth. Tenth edition. London, 1840, pp. 380.

his life been affected by the appearance of spectral figures. To such an extent did this peculiarity exist, that, if he met a friend in the street, he could not at first satisfy himself whether he saw the real or the spectral figure. By close attention he was able to perceive that the outline of the false was not quite so distinct as that of the real figure, but generally he used other means, such as touch or speech, or listening for the footsteps, to verify his visual impressions. He had also the power of calling up spectral figures at will, by directing his attention steadily to the conceptions of his own mind; and this either consisted of a figure or a scene he had witnessed, or a composition created by his imagination. But though he had the faculty of producing hallucinations, he had no power of banishing them, and, when he had once called up any particular person or scene, he could never say how long it might continue to haunt him. This gentleman was in the prime of life, of sound mind, in good health, and engaged in business. His brother was similarly affected.

Several like cases have come under the professional observation of the author. In one, the power was directly the result of attendance at spiritual meetings, and of the efforts made to become a good "medium." The patient, a lady, was of a very impressionable temperament, and was consequently well-disposed to acquire the dangerous faculty in question. At first she thought very deeply of some particular person, whose image she endeavored to form in her mind. Then she assumed that the person was really present, and she addressed conversation to him, at the same time keeping the idealistic image in her thoughts. At this period she was not deceived, for she clearly recognized the fact that the image was not present.

One day, however, she was thinking very intently of her mother, and picturing to herself her appearance as she looked when dressed for church, on a particular occasion. She was reading a book at the time, and, happening to raise her eyes, she saw her mother standing before her, clothed exactly as she had imagined her. At first she was somewhat startled, and in her agitation closed her eyes with her hands. To her surprise she still saw the phantom, but yet, not being aware of the centric origin of the image, she conceived the idea that she had really seen her mother's spirit. In a few moments it disappeared, but she soon found that she had the ability to recall it at will, and that the power existed in regard to many other forms—even those of animals, and of inanimate objects.

During the spiritualistic meetings she attended, she could thus reproduce the image of any person on whom she strongly concentrated her thoughts, and was for a long time sincere in the belief that they were real appearances. At last she lost control of the operation, and was constantly subject to hallucinations of sight and hearing. She was unable to sleep, complained of vertigo, pain in the head, and of other symptoms indicating cerebral hyperæmia. The application of ice to her head, and other suitable medication, saved her from an attack of insanity. But her nervous system was for several months in a state of exhaustion, from which she rallied with difficulty.

A young lady has recently informed me that she is able to bring visually before her the images of the characters contained in any novel she may have been recently reading, or in any striking play she may have witnessed.

It is probable that many of the visions of Jerome Cardan, and Swedenborg, were voluntary productions. On this principle can be explained many of the instances of spiritualistic hallucinations which have been detailed by inquirers willing to be deceived.

CHAPTER XIV.

FASTING GIRLS.

ANOTHER remarkable class of deceptions occasionally induced by hysteria is that embracing the "fasting girls" as they are called. They have existed for many years. Görres gives a number of examples occurring among male and female saints and other holy persons, but the records of profane history contain far more remarkable instances. Some of these may appropriately be considered in the present chapter, while others will find their proper place in that which follows. As "fasting girls" are a kind of periodical phenomenon in our own day, I shall enter at some length into the consideration of a few remarkable cases, and of the rationale of their existence.

Among these, is that of Margaret Weiss, a young girl ten years of age, who lived at Rode, a small village near Spires, and whose history has come down to us through various channels, but principally from Geraldus Bucoldianus,* who had the medical charge of her, and who wrote a little book describing his patient. Margaret is said to have abstained from all food and drink for three years, in the mean time growing, walking about, laughing, and talking like other children of her age. During the first year, however, she suffered greatly from pains

* "De puella quæ sine cibo et potu vitam transigit." Parisiis Ann. MDXLII.

in her head and abdomen, and, a common condition in hysteria—all four of her limbs were contracted. She passed neither urine nor fœces. Margaret, though only ten years old—hysteria developes the secretive faculties—played her part so well that, after being watched by the priest of the parish and Dr. Bucoldianus, she was considered free from all juggling, and was sent home to her friends by order of the King, "not," the doctor adds, "without great admiration and princely gifts." Although fully accepting the fact of Margaret's abstinence, Dr. Bucoldianus appears to have been somewhat staggered, for he asks very pertinently: "Whence comes the animal heat, since she neither eats nor drinks, and why does the body grow when nothing goes into it?"

Schenckius * quotes from Paulus Lentulus the "Wonderful History of the Fasting of Appolonia Schreira, a virgin in Berne." Lentulus states that he was with this maid on three occasions, and that, by order of the magistrate of Berne, she was taken to that city and a strict guard kept upon her. All kinds of means were set in operation to detect imposture if any existed, but none was discovered, and she was set at liberty as a genuine case of ability to live without food. In the first year of her fasting she scarcely slept, and in the second year never closed her eyes in sleep; and so she continued for a long while after.

* "*Παςατηςήσεων*, sive observationum medicarum, novarum, admirabilium et monstrasarum volumen; tomis septem de toto homine institutum." Lugduni 1606, p. 306.

These cases are cited by Wanley in his "Wonders of the Little World," but I have taken care in most instances to refer to the originals, several of which are in my library.

Schenckius also advances the case of Katharine Binder, of the Palatinate, who was closely watched by a clergyman, a statesman, and two doctors of medicine, without the detection of fraud on her part. She was said to have taken nothing but air into her system for nine years and more, as Lentulus reported on the authority of Fabricius. This last-named physician told Lentulus of another case, that of a girl fourteen years old, who certainly had taken neither food nor drink for at least three years.

"But," says Dr. Hakewel,* "the strangest that I have met with of this kind, is the history of Eve Fliegen, out of Dutch translated into English, and printed at London, *Anno* 1611, who, being born at Meurs, is said to have taken no kind of sustenance for the space of fourteen years together; that is, from the year of her age, twenty-two to thirty-six, and from the year of our Lord 1567 to 1611; and this we have confirmed by the testimony of the magistrates of the town of Meurs, as also by the minister who made trial of her in his house thirteen days together by all the means he could devise, but could detect no imposture." Over the picture of this maid, set in front of the Dutch copy, stand these Latin verses:

> "Meursæ hæc quam cernis decies ter, sexque peregit,
> Annos, bis septem prorsus non viscitur annis
> Nec potat, sic sola sedet, sic pallida vitam
> Ducit, et exigui se oblectat floribus horti."

Thus rendered in the English copy:

> "This maid of Meurs thirty and six years spent,
> Fourteen of which she took no nourishment;

---

* "Wonders of the Little World." London, 1806, p. 375.

> Thus pale and wan she sits sad and alone,
> A garden's all she loves to look upon."

Franciscus Citesius,* physician to the King of France and to Cardinal Richelieu, devotes a good deal of space and attention to the case of Joan Balaam, a native of the city of Constance. She was well grown, but of bad manners. About the eleventh year of her age she was attacked with a fever, and among other symptoms vomited for twenty days. Then she became speechless and so continued for twenty-four days. Then she talked, but her speech was raving and incoherent. Finally she lost all power of motion and of sensibility in the parts below the head and could not swallow. From thenceforth she could not be persuaded to take food. Six months afterwards she regained the use of her limbs, but the inability to swallow remained and she acquired a great loathing for all kinds of meat and drink. The secretions and excretions appeared to be arrested. Nevertheless she was very industrious, employing her time in running errands, sweeping the house, spinning, and such like. This maid continued thus fasting for the space of nearly three years, and then by degrees took to eating and drinking again.

Before coming to more recent cases, there is one other to which I desire to refer for the reason mainly that in it there was probably organic disease in addition to fraud and hysteria. It is cited by Fabricius † and by Wanley. *Anno Dom.*, 1595, a maid of about thirteen years was brought out of the dukedom

* Opuscula Medica. Parisiis, 1639, pp. 64, 65, 66.

† Observationum et curationum chirurgicæ, centuria secunda. Genevæ, 1611, p. 116.

of Juliers to Cologne, and there in a broad street at the sign of the White Horse exposed to the sight of as many as desired to see her. The parents of this maid affirmed that she had lived without any kind of food or drink for the space of three whole years; and this they confirmed by the testimony of divers persons, such as are worthy of credit. Fabricius observed her with great care. She was of a sad and melancholy countenance; her whole body was sufficiently fleshy except only her belly, which was compressed so as that it seemed to cleave to her back-bone. Her liver and the rest of her bowels were perceived to be hard by laying the hand on the belly. As for excrements, she voided none; and did so far abhor all kinds of food, that when one, who came to see her privately, put a little sugar in her mouth she immediately swooned away. But what was most wonderful was, that this maid walked up and down, played with other girls, danced, and did all other things that were done by girls of her age; neither had she any difficulty of breathing, speaking or crying out. Her parents declared that she had been in this condition for three years.

A great many more to the same effect might be adduced, but the foregoing are sufficient to indicate the fact that belief in the possibility of such occurrences was quite general, and that if doubt did exist in regard to their real nature, it was not so strong as not readily to be overcome by the tricks and devices of hysterical women.

In the following instances of more modern date the reader will perceive the view which is taken of them by physicians of the present day, and will doubtless discover their real nature.

About sixty-five years ago, a woman of Sudbury, in Staffordshire, England, named Ann Moore, declared that she did not eat, and a number of persons volunteered to watch her, in order to ascertain whether or not she was speaking the truth. The watch was continued for three weeks and then the watchers, as in other instances, reported that Ann Moore was a real oase of abstinence from food of all kinds. The Bible was always kept open on Ann's bed. Her emaciation was so extreme that it was said her vertebral column could be felt through the abdominal walls. This sad condition was asserted to have been caused by her washing the linen of a person affected with ulcers. From that time she experienced a dislike for food, and even nausea at the sight or mention of it.

As soon as the watchers reported in favor of the genuineness of Ann's pretensions her notoriety increased, and visitors came from all parts of the country, leaving donations to the extent of two hundred and fifty pounds in the course of two years. Doubts, however, again arose, and, bold from the immunity she had experienced from the first investigation, Ann in an evil moment, for the continuance of her fraud, consented to a second watching. This committee was composed of notable persons, among them being Sir Oswald Mosley, Bart., Rev. Legh Richmond, Dr. Fox, and his son, and many other gentlemen of the country. Two of them were always in her room night and day. At the suggestion of Mr. Francis Fox, the bedstead, bedding, and the woman in it were placed on a weighing machine, and thus it was ascertained that she regularly lost weight daily. At the expiration of the ninth day of this strict watching, Dr. Fox found her evidently sinking and told her she would soon die unless she took food. After a little prevarication, the woman signed a written confession that she was an impostor, and had "occasionally taken sustenance for the last six years." She also stated that during the first watch of three weeks her daughter had contrived, when washing her face, to feed her every morning, by using towels made very wet with gravy, milk, or strong arrowroot gruel, and had also conveyed food from mouth to mouth in kissing her, which it is presumed she did very often.*

In a clinical lecture delivered at St. George's Hospital,† Dr. John W. Ogle calls attention to the simulation of fasting as a manifestation of hysteria, and relates the following amusing case:

A girl strongly hysterical, aged twenty, in spite of all persuasion and medical treatment, refused every kind of food, or if made to eat, soon vomited the contents of the stomach. On November 6th, 1869, whilst the girl was apparently suffering in the same manner, the Queen passed the hospital on her way to open Blackfriars bridge. She arose in bed so as to look out of the window, although up to this time declaring that every movement of her body caused intense pain. On December 29, the following letter in the girl's handwriting, addressed to another patient in the same ward, was picked up from the floor: 'My Dear Mrs. Evens,—I was very sorry you should take the trouble of cutting me such a nice piece of bread and butter, yesterday. I would of taken it but all of them saw you send

* Wonderful Characters: By Henry Wilson and James Caulfield. London.

† British Medical Journal, July 16, 1870.

it, and then they would have made enough to have talked about. But I should be very glad if you would cut me a nice piece of crust and put it in a piece of paper and send it, or else bring it, so that they do not see it, for they all watch me very much, and I should like to be your friend and you to be mine. Mrs. Winslow, (the nurse) is going to chapel. I will make it up with you when I can go as far. Do not send it if you cannot spare it. Good bye, and God bless you.' Although she prevaricated about this letter, she appears to have gradually improved from this time on, and one day walked out of the hospital and left it altogether. She subsequently wrote a letter to the authorities expressing her regret at having gone on as she did.

One of the most remarkable instances of the kind, is that of Sarah Jacob, known as the "Welsh Fasting Girl," and whose history and tragical death excited a great deal of comment in the medical and lay press in Great Britain a few years ago. The following account of the case is mainly derived from Dr. Fowler's * interesting work.

Sarah Jacob was born May 12th, 1857. Her parents were farmers and were uneducated, simple minded, and ignorant persons. In her earlier years she had been healthy, was intelligent, given to religious reading, and was said to have written poetry of her own composition. She was a very pretty child and was, according to the testimony of the vicar, the Rev. Evan Jones, a "good girl."

* A complete History of the Welsh Fasting Girl (Sarah Jacob,) with Comments thereon, and Observations on Death from Starvation. London, 1871.

About February 15th, 1867, when she was not quite ten years of age, she complained of pain in the pit of the stomach, and one morning on getting up, she told her mother that she had found her mouth full of bloody froth. The pain continued, and medical attendance was obtained. Soon afterwards she had strong convulsions of an epileptiform character and then other spasms of a clearly hysterical form, during which her body was bent in the form of a bow as in tetanus, the head and heels only touching the bed. Then the muscular spasm ceased and she fell at full length on the bed. For a whole month she continued in a state of unconsciousness, suffering from frequent repetitions of severe convulsive attacks, during which time she took little food. Mr. Davies, the surgeon, said in his evidence, that she was for a whole month, in a kind of permanent fit, lying on her back, with rigidity of all the muscles. For some time her life was despaired of, then her fits ceased to be convulsive and consisted of short periods of loss of consciousness with sudden awakings. For the next two or three months (till August, 1867) she took daily, from six, gradually decreasing to four, teacupfuls of rice and milk, or oatmeal and milk, which according to her father's account, was cast up again immediately and blood and froth with it. During this time the bowels were only acted on once in six or nine days. "Up to this time," said her father, "she could move both arms and one leg, but the other leg was rigid."

By the beginning of October, 1867, her quantity of daily food had, it was affirmed, dwindled down to nothing but a little apple about the size of a pill, which she took from a tea-spoon. At this time she made water about every other day; she looked very bad in the face, but was not thin. On the tenth day of October, it was solemnly declared that she ceased to take any food whatever, and so continued till the day of her death, December 17th, 1869, a period of two years, two months, and one week.

"Of the veracity of the assertion in respect of *the one week*," says Dr. Fowler, "there is unfortunately plenty of evidence. To the absurdity of believing in the barest possibility of twenty-six months absolute abstinence, it is sufficient to reply that when to our knowledge, she was completely deprived of food, the girl died! The parents most persistently impressed upon every private as well as official visitor, both before and during the last fatal watching, that the girl did not take food; that she could not swallow; that whenever food was mentioned to her she became as it were, excited; that when it was offered to her she would have a fit, or the offer would make her ill. The sworn testimony of the vicar, the Rev. Wm. Thomas, Sister Clinch, Anne Jones, and the other nurses, is sufficiently confirmative on this point. Furthermore, the parents went so far as to expressly forbid the mere mention of food in the girl's presence."

Towards the end of October, 1867, the case had attracted so much attention that the inhabitants in the neighborhood first began visiting the marvellous little girl.

"In the beginning of November of the same year, the Rev. Evan Jones, B.D., the vicar of the Parish, was sent for by the parents to visit Sarah Jacob. He was at once—by the mother—told of the girl's wonderful fasting powers; it was admitted she took water occasionally. He was also informed of the extraordinary perversion of her natural functions (the suppression of urine and fœcal evacuations.) He found her lying on her back in bed, which was covered with books. There was nothing then remarkable about her dress. The girl looked weak and delicate, though not pale, and answered only in monosyllables. 'The mother said her child was very anxious about the state of her soul, that it had such an effect upon her mind that she could not sleep.' I asked her myself if she had a desire to become a member of the Church of England? She said 'Yes!' She continued to express that wish until July, 1869. At this time the reverend gentleman did not believe in the statements relative to the girl's abstinence. "Every time" he says, "that I had a conversation with her up to the end of 1868, the parents both persisted that she lived without food, and continued their statements in January and February, 1869. I remonstrated with them and dwelt upon the apparent impossibility of the thing. They still persisted that it was a fact."

"Even as late as September, 1869, the vicar reiterated his ministerial remonstrances. When, in the beginning of the spring of 1869, he observed the fantastical changes the parents made in the girl's daily attire, he told them about the remarks made in the papers about this dressing and dwelt upon the impropriety of it. They replied, 'She had no other pleasure—they did not like denying it to her.' During the following summer, finding that the girl looked more plump in the face and that her general improvement was more conspicuous, he said, 'Sarah is evidently improving and gaining, and you say she takes no food; you are certainly imposing on the public.' I then dwelt on the sinfulness of continuing the fraud on the public. I said there were on record several cases of alleged fasting, some of which had been put to the test and had been discovered to be impositions; that those families would ever be held in execration by posterity, and such would be the case with them whenever this imposture was found out. The mother then assured me no imposition would be discovered in that house, because there was none."

The father and mother both said that the Lord provided for her in a most natural way, and that it was a miracle. The father always talked about the "Doctor Mawr," meaning God Almighty; that she was supported by that "Big Doctor."

Then soon began the custom of leaving money or other presents with the child, till at last every one who visited her, was expected to give something. Open house was kept and pilgrims came from near and far to see the wonderful girl who lived without food.

When money was not forthcoming, presents of clothes, finery, books, or flowers, appear to have been substituted. Advantage was taken of these presents to bedeck the child in every variety of smartness. At one time she had a victorine about her neck and a wreath about her hair, then again, ornaments and a jacket on, and her hair neatly dressed with ribbons. At another time she had a silk shawl, a victorine around her neck, a small crucifix attached to a necklace, and little ribbons above the wrists. She had drab gloves on and her bed was nearly covered with books.

Notwithstanding the alleged fasting, Sarah Jacob continued to improve in health.

And now comes an astounding feature of this most remarkable case. The vicar became convinced that the instance was one of real abstinence. A little hysterical girl twelve years of age, by her perseverance in lying, had actually succeeded in inducing an educated gentleman to accept the truth of her statements! The following letter which was published on the 19th of February, 1869, speaks for itself:—

"A STRANGE CASE.

"To the Editor of the *Welshman*.

"Sir: Allow me to invite the attention of your readers to a most extraordinary case. Sarah Jacob, a little girl twelve years of age, and daughter of Mr. Evan Jacob, Lletherneuadd, in this parish, has not partaken of a single grain of any kind of food whatever, during the last sixteen months. She did occasionally swallow a few drops of water during the first few months of this period; but now she does not even do that. She still looks pretty well in the face and continues in the possession of all her mental faculties. She is in this and several other respects, a wonderful little girl.

"Medical men persist in saying that the thing is quite impossible, but all the nearest neighbors, who are thoroughly acquainted with the circumstances of the case, entertain no doubt whatever of the subject, and I am myself of the same opinion.

"Would it not be worth their while for medical men to make an investigation into the nature of this strange case? Mr. Evan Jacob would readily admit into his house any respectable person who might be anxious to watch it and to see for himself.

"I may add, that Lletherneuadd is a farm-house about a mile from New Inn, in this parish.

"Yours faithfully,

"THE VICAR OF LLANFIHANGEL–AR–ARTH."

The suggestions of the vicar relative to an investigation, were soon after afterwards acted upon by certain gentlemen of the neighborhood. A public meeting was called and a committee of watchers was appointed to be constantly in attendance in the room with Sarah Jacob, and to observe to the best of their ability, whether or not she took any food during the investigation. It was agreed that the watching was to continue for a fortnight.

Prior to the beginning of this watching, no precautions were taken against food being conveyed into the room and concealed there. The parents actually debarred the watchers from touching the child's bed. The very first element of success was therefore denied, and no wonder that the whole affair was subsequently regarded as an absurdity. The watching consisted in two different men taking alternate watches from eight till eight. The watching to see whether the child partook of food, commenced on March 22d, and ended April 5th, 1869—a period of fourteen days.

"During the above fortnight, one of the watchers, in turn, was always close to her bed, and in her sight day and night, and at the time the bed was being made, which was generally every other morning, the four persons were always present and had every article thoroughly examined. The parents were allowed to go near the bed, as also was the little sister, six years old, who had been Sarah's constant companion and bed-fellow.

"On Wednesday, April 7th, 1869, a public meeting was held at the Eagle Inn, Llandyfeil, to hear the statements of the parents and of the several persons who had watched the child during the fourteen days. The parents briefly detailed the condition and symptoms of their daughter from the commencement of her illness. At no time during the whole fourteen days did the pulse ever reach above ninety per minute, although exceedingly changeable, as it always had been. The following evidence was received from the watchers, and it is *said* that their statements were duly verified on oath before a magistrate:—

Watcher No. 1 said: I, Evan Edward Smith, watched Sarah Jacob for two consecutive nights, (*i. e.*, nights 22d and 23d of March) at the request of Mr. H. H. Davies, surgeon. The parents gave every facility to investigate the matter. I watched her with all possible care, and found nothing to suspect that food or drink was given her by foul means. I am quite sure she had nothing during my watch. I was dismissed on account of being suspected to doze on the second night.

Watcher No. 2. This watcher watched Sarah Jacob for a whole fortnight, and found no indications that the child had anything to eat or drink. He was a college student, Daniel Harris Davies.

Watcher No. 3. John Jones, a shopkeeper, gave similar evidence. He was a decided sceptic before he began watching, but after twelve days was thoroughly convinced of the fact that nothing in the shape of nourishment was given to the poor child. He watched every movement of all the inmates, and found nothing that would lead him to suspect that any nourishment was given to the little girl.

Watcher No. 4. James Harris Davies, a medical student, spoke in like manner, and was perfectly positive that nothing had been given to her during the fortnight he had watched there, with the exception of three drops of water, once, to moisten her lips with. He was as great a sceptic as any one before he began watching, but as he saw nothing to confirm his suspicions, he could conscientiously say that nothing had been given her during his watch.

Watcher No. 5. Evan Davies, of Powel Castle, who only watched her for one day, gave similar evidence, but as he was a neighbour he was dismissed for a stranger.

Watcher No. 6. Herbert Jones, watched only one day, and spoke in a similar manner, and was dismissed on account of his credulity.

Watcher No. 7. Thomas Davies, who had been the greatest sceptic of all, was strongly convinced. He watched Sarah Jacob twelve days, and was quite positive that nothing could have been given her during his watch. He watched her with all possible care, and was very cautious to be in a prominent place, where Sarah Jacob's mouth was always in sight.

Evidence, however, was given which went to show that the watching was very imperfectly performed; that occasionally the watchers left before their time had expired; that intoxicating liquors were taken by them to the house, and that one of them was drunk while there. It was also shown that the father and mother had free access to the bed, while the watchers were absolutely prohibited from examining it. It is therefore with entire justification that Dr. Fowler states that the watching "was the greatest possible farce and mockery."

After the report of the watchers the notoriety of Sarah Jacob of course became still greater; crowds came to visit her, and among others the Rev. Frederic Rowland Young went to see her, and made an unsuccessful effort to cure her by laying on of hands. When Dr. Fowler visited her, August 30th, 1869, on getting out at the nearest railway station, he was met by little boys bearing placards with the words "Fasting Girl," and "This is the shortest way to Llethernoryadd-ucha," on them. In his letter to the *Times*, giving an account of his visit, Dr. Fowler says:—

"The first impression was most unfavorable, and to a medical man the appearances were most suspicious. The child was lying on a bed decorated as a bride, having around her head a wreath of flowers, from which was suspended a smart ribbon, the ends of which were joined by a small bunch of flowers, after the present fashion of ladies' bonnet strings. Before her, at proper reading distance, was an open Welsh book, supported by two other books on her body. The blanket covering was clean, tidy, and perfectly smooth. Across the fire-place, which was nearly opposite the foot of her bed, was an arrangement of shelves, well stocked with English and Welsh books, the gifts of various visitors to the house. The child is thirteen years of age, and is undoubtedly very pretty. Her face was plump, and her cheeks and lips of a beautiful rosy color. Her eyes were bright and sparkling, the pupils were very dilated, in a measure explicable by the fact of the child's head and face being shaded from the window-light by the projecting side of the cupboard bedstead. There was that restless movement and frequent looking out at the corners of the eyes so characteristic of simulative disease. Considering the lengthened inactivity of the girl, her muscular development was very good, and the amount of fat layer not inconsiderable. My friend stated that she looked even better than she did about a twelvemonth ago. There was a slight perspiration over the surface of the body. The pulse was perfectly natural, as were also the sounds of the lungs and heart, so far as I was enabled to make a stethoscopic examination. Having received permission to do this, I proceeded to make the necessary derangement of dress, when the girl went off into what the mother called a fainting fit. This consisted of nothing but a little and momentary hysterical crying and sobbing. The color never left the lips or cheeks. The pulse remained of the same power. Consciousness could have been but slightly diminished, inasmuch as on my then opening the eyelids I perceived a distinct upward and other movement of the eyeballs. Each percussion stroke of my examination, and even the pressure of the stethoscope, produced an expression of pain, which elicited a natural sympathy from the mother, and an assertion that a continuance of such examination would bring on further fits. On percussing the region of the stomach, I most distinctly perceived the sound of gurgling, which we know to be caused by the admixture of air and fluid in motion. The most positive assertion of the parents was subsequently made that saving a fortnightly moistening of her lips with cold water, the child had neither ate nor drank anything for the last twenty-three months. The whole region of the belly was tympanitic, and the muscular walls of this cavity were tense and drum-like—a condition not infrequently concomitant of a well-known class of nervous disorders. The child's intellectual faculties and special senses were perfectly healthy. Before her illness she was very much devoted to religious reading. This devotion has lately considerably increased. She is a member of the Church of England, and has been confirmed."

Dr. Fowler then adds some other interesting particulars, all going to show the impossibility of the girl's being the subject of any exhausting disease, or of even having been continuously in bed, as her parents asserted, for nearly two years; and then says:—

"The whole case is in fact one of simulative hysteria, in a young girl having the propensity to deceive very strongly developed. Therewith may be probably associated the power or habit of prolonged fasting. Both patient and mother admitted the occasional occurrence of the choking sensation called *globus hystericus*.

This letter excited renewed discussion in the newspapers, and a second public meeting was called to make arrangements for a second watching. At this meeting it was decided to bring down from Guy's Hospital, London, several trained nurses, who were to conduct the watching; and the following resolutions were adopted, as expressing the terms under which the inquiry was to be conducted:—

1. It would be advisable, before taking any steps in the matter, to obtain a written legal guarantee from the father of Sarah Jacob sanctioning the necessary proceedings. 2. That the duty of the nurses shall be to watch Sarah Jacob with a

view to ascertain whether she partakes of any kind of food, and at the end of a fortnight to report upon the case before the local committee in Carmarthenshire, and, if required, at Guy's Hospital. 3. That two nurses shall be constantly awake and on the watch in the girl's room, night and day. 4. It would be advisable for the nearest medical practitioner to watch the progress of the case; and it will be absolutely necessary for him to *be prepared against any serious symptoms of exhaustion, supervening on the strict enforcement of the watching, and to act according to his judgment.* 5. That the room in which the girl sleeps shall be bared of all unnecessary furniture, and all possible places in the room for the concealment of food shall be closed and kept under the continual scrutiny of the watchers. 6. That if considered desirable by the local medical practitioner, or by the nurses, the bedstead on which the girl now lies shall be replaced by a single iron one. 7. That the bed on which the parents now sleep, in Sarah Jacob's room, shall be given up absolutely to the nurses. 8. That the parents be not allowed to sleep in the same room as the girl; that if they cannot at all times be prevented from approaching her, they should be previously searched (their pockets and other recesses of clothing as well as the interior of their mouths); and that no wetted towels or other such articles be allowed to be used about the girl by the parents, or any other person save the nurses; that the children of the family, and in fact every other person whatever (except the nurses), have similar restraints put upon them. 9. That the nurses have the sole management of preparing the room, bed, and patient, prior to the commencement of the watching. 10. That, as it is asserted the action of the bowels and bladder is entirely suspended, special attention must be directed to these organs.

Four experienced women nurses were accordingly deputed from Guy's Hospital to take the entire charge of Sarah Jacob, and to watch her for fourteen days. They were instructed not to prevent her having food if she asked for it, but they were to see that she got none without their knowledge. On the 9th of December, 1869, at 4 p.m., the room was cleared of people and the watching began.

In the first place it was ascertained that the girl had repeated evacuations of urine, and once, at least, of fœces.

Gradually evidences of mental and physical disturbance began to appear. The watch was so closely kept that no food or drink reached the child, and she did not ask for any.

"At 10 P. M.," to quote the language of the journal kept by the sister nurse, "she was restless and threw her arms about. She was very cold, and the nurses put warm flannels on her. This was the last day on which she passed urine.

Thursday, December 16, 3 A. M.—She was rolling from one side of the bed to the other. At half-past three she wished the bed made, and they made it. She was looking very pale and anxious. Her eyes were sunk and her nose pinched, and the cheek bones were prominent. Her arms and hands were cold, her feet and legs were the same. Ann Jones, one of the nurses, says in her memoranda, "She was very restless and appeared to me to be sinking. Her lips were very dry, and her mouth seemed parched." The peculiar smell (the starvation smell) about the bed was so strong as to make the sister nurse quite ill.

At 11 A. M., the vicar saw her and told the parents that the child was gradually failing, and suggested to them the propriety of sending the nurses away and giving her a chance to obtain food, but they refused, saying that there was nothing to do but what the nurses were doing, and that they had seen her quite as weak before. The parents were urged by others to give up the fight by sending the nurses away, but they refused on the ground that want of food had nothing to do with the symptoms, and that she would not eat whether the nurses were there or not.

Ann Jones subsequently testified before the coroner: "Before one and two o'clock on Thursday afternoon (Dec. 16), she kept talking to herself. I could not understand whether she was speaking Welsh or English. Up to that time I could understand her. She pointed her fingers at some books; I gave her one, but she took no notice of it; she was not able to read it. *Both parents were then told the girl was dying.*"

Repeatedly they were begged to withdraw the nurses, and again and again they refused, saying there was no occasion—that she had often been in that way, that it was not from want of food, etc. The girl became weaker and weaker; low, muttering delirium ensued, and on the 17th of December, 1869, at about half-past three o'clock, P.M., the "Welsh Fasting Girl" died, actually starved to death, in the middle of the nineteenth century and in one of the most Christian and civilized countries of the world!

But this was not the end. Public opinion was much excited both against those who had sanctioned and conducted what appeared to have been a senseless and cruel experiment, and against the father and mother who had wilfully and persistently refused to allow food to be given to the dying child. A coroner's inquest was held, and the coroner appears to have made a very satisfactory charge to the jury after the rendition of the testimony. He said there could be no doubt of the child having died of starvation, and that the responsibility rested with the father, who had knowingly and designedly failed to cause his child to take food. The mother was not responsible unless it could be shown that she had been given food for the child by the father, and had withheld it from her. It was marvellous, he said, how the father could have made out such a story—such a hideous mass of nonsense, as he had under oath attempted to impose on the jury.

The jury deliberated for a quarter of an hour, and then returned a verdict of "Died from starvation, caused by negligence to induce the child to take food on the part of the father;" which constituted manslaughter.

Evan Jacob was therefore arrested. But the Secretary of State for the Home Department took the matter up and determined that the proceedings should go farther than the local authorities intended. At first it was contemplated to indict the members of the General Committee for conspiracy, but it was finally concluded to include only the medical gentlemen who had accepted the responsibility of superintending the watching, as well as both parents of the deceased child.

The initial proceeding took place before a full bench of magistrates, and continued eight days. The Crown and the accused had eminent counsel, and many witnesses were examined. At the conclusion of the inquiry the presiding magistrate announced that it had been determined by the court that no case had been made out against the physicians, who had not been shown to have undertaken any other duty than that of advising the nurses, and that it did not appear that their advice had been asked. As to the father and mother the court had decided to send them both for trial for manslaughter, at the next assizes. In due time they were arraigned, they pleaded not guilty, but after being defended by able counsel, the jury, after an absence of about half an hour, returned with a verdict of guilty against both the prisoners, but with a recommendation of the mother to the merciful consideration of the court, on the ground that she was under the control of her husband. The man protested his innocence, and the woman "buried her face in her shawl and wept bitterly."

His Lordship, in passing sentence, said: "Prisoners at the bar, you have been found guilty of a most aggravated offence. I entirely concur with the verdict which the jury have given, and I shall act upon the recommendation which they have presented in favor of the female prisoner, the mother, though, I must say, that I cannot but feel that it is a greater crime in the mother than the father, since it is more contrary to the common nature of mothers, to neglect their children in the manner in which you have treated this unfortunate child. It is contrary to the nature, even, of a father. But I shall act upon the recommendation of the jury, upon the ground they have put forward, that you have been subject to the control of your husband more than has appeared from the evidence of the case. But the offence is, as I have said, a serious one, on this ground; that there can be no doubt that both of you have persisted in this fraudulent deception, upon your neighbors, and upon the public, and that in order to carry out that fraudulent deception and to preserve yourselves from detection you were willing to risk the life of that child. The life of that child has been lost in that wicked experiment which you tried. Therefore, the sentence that I shall inflict on you, Evan Jacob, is, that you be imprisoned and kept at hard labor for twelve calendar months; and that upon you, Hannah Jacob, will be more lenient in consideration of the recommendation of the jury, and it is, that you be imprisoned and kept to hard labor for the period of six calendar months."

Thus ended one of the most remarkable and interesting histories of human folly, credulity, and criminality which the present day has produced. Comment upon its teaching is scarcely necessary; but the thoughtful reader will not fail to perceive how important a bearing it has upon the whole subject of belief without full and free inquiry, and that how all the facts which science has gathered during ages of painful labor, go for naught, even with educated persons, when brought face to face with the false assertions of a hysterical girl, and of two ignorant and deceitful peasants. If there is any one thing we know, it is that there can be no force without the metamorphosis of matter of some kind. Here was a girl maintaining her weight—actually growing—her animal heat kept at its due standard, her mind active, her heart beating, her lungs respiring, her skin exhaling, her limbs moving whenever she wished them to move, and all, as very many persons supposed, without the ingestion of the material by which alone such things could be. And yet such is the tendency of the average human mind to be deceived, that it would be perfectly possible to re-enact in the city of New York the whole tragedy of Sarah Jacob, should ever a hysterical girl take it into head to do so; and there would not be wanting, even from among those who might read this history, individuals who would credit any monstrous declarations she might make. Even now in a little town in Belgium, an ecstatic girl is going through the same performance with extraordinary additions, and books are written by learned physicians and theologians, with the object of establishing the truth of her pretensions. To this most remarkable instance the attention of the reader will presently be invited. But in view of these things one is almost tempted to say with Cardinal Carrafa, "*Quandoquidem populus decipi vult, decipiatur.*"

CHAPTER XV.

THE HYSTEROID AFFECTIONS—CATALEPSY, ECSTASY AND HYSTERO-EPILEPSY.

ALTHOUGH in systematic medical treatises these diseases would properly be considered separately, for the purposes of the present inquiry they may be advantageously brought together under one head. They are hysteroid without actually being hysteria. It is very often the case that they are co-existent in the same patient, or they alternate one with the other. Indeed, it is quite rare to find a case in which one of them is present, without one or both of the others being also manifested.

In all of these diseases, we have affections which are well calculated to impress ignorant and superstitious persons with a sense of mystery, and they are therefore admirably adapted to fulfil the requirements of religious enthusiasts and impostors, or of spiritualistic mountebanks.

Catalepsy is characterized by the suspension of the understanding and of sensibility, and by a tendency in the muscles to preserve for a long time any degree of contraction which may be given to them. Thus if the arm of a cataleptic patient be extended it remains so for several minutes, sometimes hours ; if the leg be raised from the bed, the muscles continue

SPIRITUALISM

AND

ALLIED CAUSES AND CONDITIONS

OF

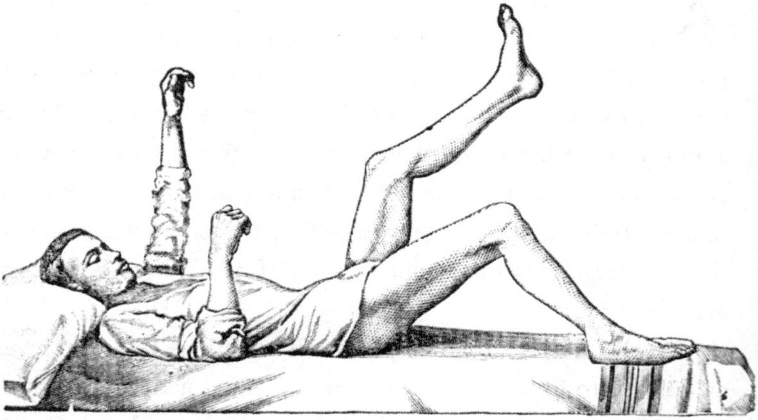

Fig. 6.

The aspect of a cataleptic patient is very striking. The eyelids are sometimes wide open, at others gently closed; the pupils are dilated and do not respond to strong light; the respiration is slow, regular, but generally so feeble as to be perceived with difficulty; the pulse is usually almost imperceptible, but is rhythmical and sluggish; the face is pale, the mouth is half open, and the rigidity of the body and the coldness of the extremities add to the death-like appearance which impresses all beholders.

The cutaneous sensibility is ordinarily completely abolished. Pins may be thrust into the skin, and they are not felt; but owing to the abolition of the power of motion and of reflex action, it is possible that in some cases at least, the patients would give some evidence of sensation if they could. Cases are on record in which tears have been caused by excessive emotional disturbance, excited by the words or actions of persons surrounding the patients; thus showing that the senses of sight and hearing were capable of being exercised. Such instances are, however, rare, and are probably imperfectly developed paroxysms, or those complicated with hysteria or ecstasy.

The paroxysm may last a few minutes or hours, or may be prolonged for several days. In a case recently under my care, one paroxysm continued, with scarcely even a remission, for eleven days. The ability to swallow was not lost—it very rarely is, and the patient was fed at regular intervals, taking what was put in her mouth and eating it, without appearing to appreciate the taste or character of the food.

In the less perfectly developed forms of the cataleptic condition, the afflicted individuals, though taking no cognizance of circumstances surrounding them, are capable of a certain exalted esoteric mental action, which passes with the vulgar for illumination, inspiration, or spiritualism. Such cases were common enough among the women of the thirteenth, fourteenth, fifteenth, and sixteenth centuries, shut up in convents, and are not infrequently met with in our own time. Chambers * cites from DeHaen, the case of a child twelve years of age, who began a paroxysm by being cataleptic, and ended by reciting the metrical Protestant version of David's Psalms, saying her catechism with proof texts, and preaching a sermon on adultery.

A young girl, recently under my professional care, was cataleptic on an average once a week, and epileptic twice or three times in the intervals. Five years previously she had spent six months in France, but had not acquired more than a very slight knowledge of the language, scarcely, in fact, sufficient to enable her to ask for what she wanted at her meals. Immediately before her cataleptic seizures, she went into a state of ecstasy, during which she recited poetry in French, and delivered harangues about virtue and godliness in the same language. She pronounced at these times exceedingly well, and seemed never at a loss for a word. To all surrounding influences she was apparently dead. But she sat bolt upright in her chair, her eyes staring at vacancy, and her organs of speech in constant action. Gradually she passed into the cataleptic paroxysm. She was an excellent example of what Mrs. Hardinge calls a "trance medium." The materialistic influence of

* Reynold's System of Mediums, p. 104; Art. Catalepsy.

bromide of potassium, however, cured her catalepsy and epilepsy, destroyed her knowledge of the French tongue and made her corporeal structure so gross that the spirits refused to make further use of it for their manifestations.

Many of the cases to which reference has already been made as being induced by emotional disturbance at camp-meetings, revivals, and other religious gatherings, were instances of catalepsy. The electro-biologist knows well the ease with which the condition can be excited by the principle of suggestion, and he therefore employs it in his public exhibitions with great effect. He renders the arms and legs of his subjects rigid, by telling them in a confident and commanding tone that they are so, and he produces the other phenomena of the cataleptic state with equal facility.

Catalepsy often exists in combination with somnambulism, either natural or artificial. In former times cataleptics were thought to be "possessed," and even in our own day, such afflicted persons are by some authorities regarded as being under demoniac influence. To this division of the subject we shall presently return.

Ecstasy, though closely allied to catalepsy, differs from it in several important particulars, among others, in the fact that the ecstatic recollects the train of thought which has been going on during the seizure, and speaks of it usually on emerging from the paroxysm. Besides, in ecstasy there is rather muscular immobility than rigidity, although this latter is sometimes present. The eyes are open, the lips parted, the face is turned upward, the hands raised as if to heaven; and the body is erect and stretched out to its utmost height, or else is extended to its full length in the recumbent position. A peculiar expression of joy lights up the face, and this is the radiance spoken of by camp-meeting and revivalist preachers, ignorant of the symptoms of the affection in question.

At times, various attitudes are assumed which are in consonance with the ideas passing through the ecstatic's mind. The body may thus be elevated on the toes, and the arms extended as if in ærial flight, or it is stretched out on the bed or floor, the feet crossed one over the other and the arms placed at right angles to the body, in the position of crucifixion.

Mr. Bourneville * cites the case of Ler., a hystero-epileptic, to whom, hereafter, fuller reference will be made, who at one time had a cruciform paroxysm. Her head was strongly thrown back; her eyelids, half open, were in continual motion; the muscles of the jaws were contracted, and those of the neck were hard and tense.

The superior extremities were extended at right angles with the trunk, the hands closed, and the fingers flexed so strongly on the palm as to render it impossible to open them.

The inferior extremities were stretched out to their full length, the sole of one foot being in contact with the dorsum of the other.

In a word, the rigidity was such that the body could have been raised from either end like a bar of iron, (Fig. 7.) The attack lasted about four hours, and then Ler. opened her eyes and recovered consciousness, exclaiming, "O, my God, I was so happy!"

Among celebrated cataleptics and ecstatics, may be men-

* Louise Lateau, etc., Paris, 1875, p. 13.

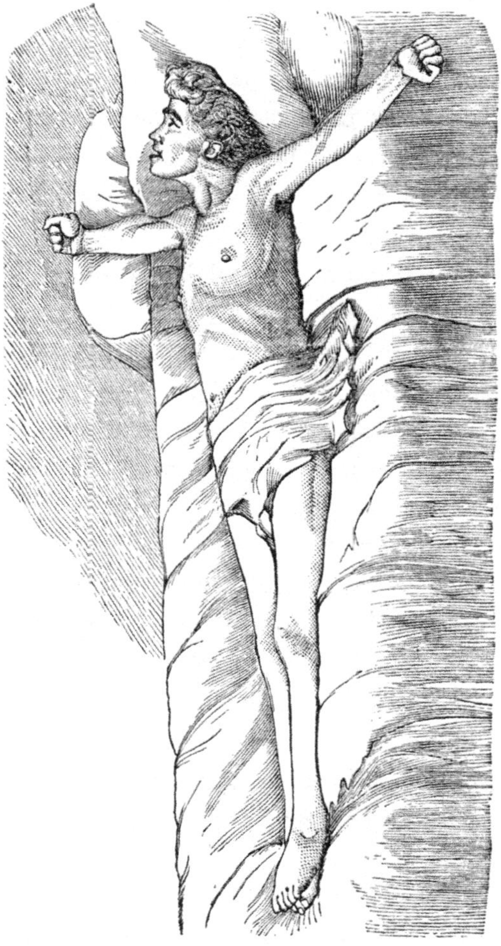

Fig. 7.

tioned Elizabeth of Hungary, St. Gertrude, St. Bridget, St. Catherine of Sienna, Joan of Arc, St. Theresa, and Madame Guyon. Others who were not only cataleptics, ecstatics, and hystero-epileptics, but who were also the subject of the stigmata, will be separately considered.

The conventual life was especially favorable to the production of all forms of catalepsy and ecstasy, and sometimes, as in the instances of the nuns of Loudun, the disorder assumed a degree of malignancy which all the powers of the Church could not abate.

It is a striking fact, which would be laughable, but for the frequently lamentable results which ensued, that while the Catholic ecstatics inveighed against the heretical sects which were springing up on all sides, and consigned them to torture and the flames, these, the Calvinists, Camisards, Pre-adamites, Jumpers, Anabaptists, Bewailers, Sanguinarians, Tremblers, etc., etc., denounced the Pope as Anti-Christ, desecrated churches and exhibited a ferocity which, in its sanguinary character, has rarely been equalled in the history of the world.

Now, as has already been remarked, in the imperfect forms of catalepsy or ecstasy, consciousness is not altogether lost. Montgeron noticed this fact, and in speaking of persons affected, says, "they generally saw those who were about them, spoke to them and heard their answers, though at the same time their minds were entirely absorbed in the contemplation of objects which a superior power enabled them to see." It must be recollected that Montgeron was a believer in the supernatural origin of these manifestations of disease. At the present day he would have been a shining light among Spiritualists.

He further observes, that in these undeveloped forms of both diseases, as noticed among the Jansenist convulsionnaires, the affected individuals appeared as if struck by the sight of some object before unseen, and the contemplation of which filled them with the most ravishing joy. They raised their eyes and their hands on high, leaped towards heaven, and seemed as if about to fly into the air. They appeared to be absorbed in the contemplation of celestial beauties. Their faces were animated with a brilliant glow, and their eyes, which could not be closed during the continuance of the ecstasy, remained open and fixed on the spiritualized object on which they gazed. They were, in a manner, transfigured; they appeared to be perfectly unlike their natural selves. Those who ordinarily were low and repulsive, were changed so profoundly that they could not be recognized.

It will be brought to mind that Mr. Wesley, in the extracts from his journal which I have cited, speaks of this change of countenance as a supernatural gift.

The following example is domestic, and is taken from the *Norfolk Beacon*, of August 19th, 1824. It was copied into other religious papers without the least doubt being expressed of its being produced by the direct and special action of the "Spirit of God."*

"A singular display of the goodness and power of Almighty God at a camp-meeting held at Tangier Island.

"Miss Narcissa Crippin, a highly-respectable young lady,

* "Observations on the Influence of Religion upon the Health and Physical Welfare of Mankind. By Almirah Brigham, M.D." Boston, 1835, p. 305.

nineteen years of age, and a zealous Christian, was, on the evening of the 15th instant, so operated on by the Spirit of God that her face became too bright and shining for mortal eyes to gaze upon without producing the most awful feeling to the beholders. It resembled the reflection of the sun upon a bright cloud. The appearance of her face for the space of forty minutes, was truly angelic, during which time she was silent, after which she spoke and expressed her happy and heavenly feelings, when her dazzling countenance gradually faded, and her face resumed its natural appearance. The writer of this paragraph was an eye-witness of the circumstance above stated —such a sight he never expected to behold with mortal eyes, and to give a true description of which would be beyond the ability of mortal man. While she remained in the situation above described, she was seen by more than two hundred persons, a few of whom have subscribed their names hereto.

"WM. LEE (Rev.),
"WM. E. WISE,
"JOHN BAYLY."

I have frequently seen this remarkable change induced in the faces of persons of both sexes. It appears to be directly due to a relaxation of all the muscles of the face concerned in expression, and is accompanied by suffusion of the eyes and dilatation of the pupils. Undoubtedly the instances mentioned in the Bible as transfigurations, (see Exodus xxxiv. 29–35; Matthew xvii. 1, 2; Mark ix. 2, 3; Luke ix. 29) were of this character.

Almost fifty years ago, a very remarkable case of preaching-ecstasy, or, as it would now be called by some, trance-medium ship, occurred in this city in the person of a maiden lady, of delicate health, named Rachel Baker. Dr. S. L. Mitchill took great interest in her case, and had her sermons reported by a stenographer, and published. Miss Baker was the daughter of a respectable farmer in Onondaga County, New York, and had received a plain but substantial education. About the age of twenty, she became much exercised on the subject of religion, and at length her mind became seriously affected, and she fell into the habit of trance-preaching. Her parents were at first impressed at what they regarded as a most extraordinary gift, though they afterward became convinced that it was the result of disease, and accordingly brought her to the city of New York, in order that she might have the benefit of the best medical skill. Crowds flocked to hear her preach at the houses of different medical practitioners. Her discourses were highly respectable in point of style and arrangement, and were interspersed with Scripture quotations. After her health was restored, she lost the faculty of trance-preaching and never regained it. She died in 1843.*

But ecstatics and cataleptics do other things fully as remarkable as trance-preaching. The performances of the Jansenist convulsionnaires have already been alluded to, but they are so various in their character, that there is scarcely a subject connected with paroxysms of disturbed mobility and sensibility, with which some of them are not *en rapport*.

Among them was a woman, or rather a girl, Marie Sonet, who, on account of her apparent incombustibility, was called

* Remarkable sermons of Rachel Baker and Pious Ejaculations delivered during sleep, taken down in short hand, etc. London, 1815.

the salamander. We have seen what Mr. Home has done in the way of showing his ability to resist heat; the salamander was immeasurably his superior. Let us begin with a certificate which was published at the time:

"We, the undersigned, François Desvernays, priest, doctor of theology of the house and society of the Sorbonne; Pierre Jourdan, licentiate of the Sorbonne, Canon of Bayeux; Lord Edmund de Rumond, of Perth; Louis Bazile Carré de Montgeron, Counsellor to the Parliament; Armand Arouet, Treasurer of the Chamber of Accounts; Alexandre Robert Boindin, Esquire; [and five others;] certify that we have this day, between the hours of eight and ten o'clock in the evening, seen Marie Sonet while in convulsion, her head on one stool and her feet on another, the said stools being entirely within a large fire-place and under the mantel-piece, so that her body was in the air above the fire, which burned with extreme violence, remaining in that position for thirty-six minutes in four different times, (nine minutes each time) without the cloth in which she was wrapped (she was without other clothes) being burned, although the flames sometimes extended above her—the which appears to us to be quite supernatural.

"Again, we certify that while we were signing the present certificate, the said Sonet placed herself over the fire in the manner previously described, and remained there nine minutes, appearing to sleep above the brazier, which was very hot, having been replenished with fifteen large logs, and a faggot of kindling wood, during the last two hours and a quarter. In testimony of which," etc., [here follow the signatures.]

The Abbé Asfeld, who wrote against the Jansenists, thus

describes what he saw: "Sonet went behind a screen and was there divested of all her clothing, except her chemise and a little jacket. Then she was entirely wrapped up in a cloth, which was fastened with strong pins." To this Carré de Montgeron replies, "It is not true that she was reduced to a chemise and a jacket; she had besides, a corset, a petticoat, and stockings." "Then," continues the Abbé Asfeld, "being thus enamelled, she called for the stools, and immediately two of the brethren brought them and placed them *near the fire-place*, where there was a good fire. Sonet placed herself on them, and from this performance she has received the name of 'Salamander.'" To this Carré de Montgeron rejoins, "One would think, from this account, that the stools were placed opposite the fire. Now, it is a fact which has been witnessed a number of times by many persons, that at each representation the two stools, which were of iron, except two boards on which Sonet supported her head and feet, were placed in the fire-place on each side, so that when the girl was on them she was immediately over the flames, and so that no matter how great the fire was, she suffered no inconvenience therefrom, nor was the cloth in which she was wrapped even singed, although it was often in the midst of the flames." And he pushed his adversary so hard that the Abbé had to admit that ordinarily the *convulsionnaire remained long enough in the fire for a piece of beef, mutton, or veal, to be roasted!* *

Marie Sonet was not the only "incombustible." Many others appeared, the example she afforded spreading, like other

* Mathieu. "Histoire des Miraculés et des Convulsionnaires de Saint Médard." Paris, 1864, p. 262, et seq.

hysterical performances, by contagion. Of course Marie Sonet and her imitators did not expose their unprotected persons to the fire, and we have already seen how the necessary immunity can be obtained. The cloth in which she was so securely enveloped was of incombustible material, or rendered fire-proof by some one of the preparations to which reference has already been made.

But this was not all. There was one Charlotte Laporte, called the "Sucker," whose proceedings were so disgusting that it is with hesitation I mention them. We must, however, re member with Bacon that: "*Quidquid essentia dignum est, id etiam scientia dignum.*" The fact that such things could be, is my excuse for bringing them forward in illustration of the occasional depravity of the human mind, even when actuated by noble impulses. The "Sucker," then, went about claiming to cure ulcers, cancers, and other open sores, by sucking them while in a state of ecstasy. She, also, had her imitators—women all. They applied their tongues and lips to the most disgusting ulcers, full of pus and horrible to see, and sucked them till they were perfectly clean. They even swallowed the fœtid exudations with impunity and even relish. They washed the dressings which had been applied to such sores, and then drank the water!

These people were heretics, but such vile actions are not confined to those who are heterodox in religious faith. Thus we read in Görres* that so great was the holiness of St. Catherine of Sienna that she did some things that were almost incredible. There was a widow named Teeta who, on account of her poverty, lived in a hospital. But her body was covered

* Op. cit., t. I., p. 277.

entirely with a hideous leprosy, and she was required to quit not only the hospital, but the city, because she was an object of horror to everybody. Catherine, however, took care of her, and with admirable charity dressed her sores. The woman, however, was puffed up with pride, and treated her nurse in the most haughty and overbearing manner. Nevertheless, Catherine continued her cares, and even contracted the leprosy in consequence of the frequent contacts with this woman. The latter died, as was very proper, and Catherine laid out the body. She had her reward, as was also proper—for if the story be true, she had acted with tender charity—for her hands immediately became free from leprosy.

So far, so good; but she went farther. There was another woman who had a cancer of the breast, from which the odor was such that no one could remain near her, and she had great difficulty in getting the attention she required. Catherine, however, assumed the charge and cleansed the sore, with a cheerful face, to the great astonishment of the woman herself. But it was really so disgusting that one day the stomach of Catherine revolted. Indignant against herself, she said to her body: How! Thou hast a horror of thy sister, baptized, as thou hast been, in the blood of our Lord! I will pay thee up! Saying which she applied her mouth, her nose and her whole face to the disgusting wound, and kept them there till she felt that her soul had conquered the repugnance of the flesh. Nevertheless, the virgin had at times her moments of loathing. "And then," says Görres, "she did what perhaps no one had ever done before her—she drank the pus and the filthy discharges which she had sucked from the wound. She subsequently declared to her confessor that she had never drank in all her life a more agreeable beverage." We see, therefore, that four hundred years before Charlotte Laporte began her horrible operations, there was a proto-sucker in the person of one of the most worthy saints of the Calendar.

MM. Mauriac and Verdalle* give a very interesting account of an ecstatic woman, who daily enacted the passion of Jesus, terminating in the usual manner in the crucifixion. This woman, Berguille, had been of good health till, in 1871, she lost one of her children. A short time afterward she began to have visions of her child every night, and then she was seized with obstinate vomitings, which were only cured by drinking the water of Lourdes, ordinary therapeutics not having been very efficacious.

In a short time she began to have paroxysms of ecstasy. In these, there were more or less profound abolition of sensibility, general and special, and hallucinations of various kinds. At first these seizures were at no fixed intervals of time, but after a while they occurred regularly on Friday and in the afternoon. The duration was in the beginning only a few minutes, but latterly they got to lasting several hours.

Like many other ecstatics, Berguille was devoted to making predictions both in religion and politics. Unfortunately for her reputation, nothing that she foretold ever came to pass. Thus, on the 26th of July, 1873, she said, "The great king, the most Christian king, promised to France, will come very soon. He is Monseigneur the Count de Chambord." On the 24th of August: "The three days of darkness are near; terrible events

* Etude Médicale sur l'extatique de Fontet. Paris, 1875.

are about to take place. Paris will be entirely destroyed." On the 11th of September Berguille declared that "The great King Henry V. will come, not by the votes of men, but by the will of the all-powerful God, and because it is necessary for him to save France."

When visited by MM. Mauriac and Verdalle, Berguille was lying in bed. She is described as a woman of about forty-five years of age, brown complexion, muscles and limbs well developed, but without much fat, eyes blue, widely open and staring vaguely. She smiled kindly when questions were put to her, and answered with sufficient intelligence.

On being asked why she was in bed, she answered that she was in pain night and day; and when requested to state where she felt the pain, she answered the backs and palms of her hands, the tops and soles of her feet, and the right side. These places were in correspondence with the five wounds of Christ, but the pain in the side, she had on the right, while other ecstatics, as Louise Lateau, had it on the left. The miracle-believers ought to find it difficult to reconcile a discrepancy like this.

Relative to her visions and what she heard during her ecstasies, she said that she saw Jesus Christ in His passion, that she heard voices, but she could not repeat what was told her. Her pulse was from 68 to 72.

At about one o'clock the ecstasy began. Her pulse rose to 80. She clasped her hands over her heart, her gaze became fixed, her eyes were widely opened, her lips moved as though she was muttering prayers, and there were frequent movements of deglutition. Her pupils were slightly dilated, but contracted when a light was brought to them. Her limbs were rigid, but it was noticed that she flexed them very readily when she altered her position a little or arranged her dress. In a few minutes she raised herself somewhat awkwardly on her knees, her hands still being clasped and her eyes fixed. Then began the passion on the way to the cross, during which she walked on her knees around the bed, changing her position twelve times and falling three times in the traditional manner. To make this journey, required thirty-six minutes, and this done the next act, the crucifixion, was in order.

Suddenly she threw herself back on the bed, extended her arms from each side, and remained immovable. The pulse was 112, the respirations 100. The muscles of the chest seemed to be paralyzed, only the diaphragm acting. The eyes were closed.

The limbs were in a state of forced extension and very rigid; the cutaneous sensibility to pinching, pricking, and to the electrical stimulus was abolished. The latter, a very strong induced current, caused muscular contractions, but no sensation. There was not the least flinching. Things went on in this way for over three hours, and then she sang the "*Salve Regina*," exclaimed "Oh, what sorrow!" and gradually recovered her senses.

We have seen how greatly a weak, hysterical girl can disturb the community in which she lives. The history of the world is full of examples, in which whole nations and groups of nations have been so deeply influenced by ecstatics of both sexes, as to have their entire political status changed thereby.

The instance of Joan of Arc has already been cited. It is interesting to quote her own touching and evidently sincere words, detailing how she was led to take the leadership of the armies of France, and conduct them on to victory.

"It is now seven years ago," she said to her judges, "on a summer's day, towards the middle hour, I was about thirteen years of age, and in my father's garden—that I heard for the first time on my right hand, towards the church, a voice, and there stood a figure in a bright radiance before my eyes. It had the appearance and look of a right good and virtuous man, bore wings, was surrounded with light on all sides, and by the angels of heaven. It was the Archangel Michael. The voice seemed to me to command respect; but I was yet a child, and was frightened at the figure, and doubted very much whether it were the Archangel. I saw him and the angels as distinctly before my eyes as I now see you, my judges." With words of encouragement the Archangel announces to her that God had taken pity upon France, and that she must hasten to the assistance of the King. At the same time he promised her that St. Catherine and St. Margaret would soon visit her; he told her that she should do what they commanded her, because they were sent by God to guide and conduct her. "Upon this," continued Joan, "St. Catherine and St. Margaret appeared to me, as the Archangel had foretold. They ordered me to get ready to go to Robert de Baudricourt, the King's captain. He would several times refuse me, but at length would consent, and give me people who would conduct me to the King. Then should I raise the siege of Orleans. I replied to them that I was a poor child, who understood nothing about riding on horseback and making war. They said I should carry my banner with courage; God would help me, and win back for my King his entire kingdom. As soon as I knew that I was to proceed on this errand, I avoided as much as I could taking part in the sports and amusements of my young companions. So have the Saints conducted me during seven years, and have given me support and assistance in all my needs and labors, and now no day goes by but they come to see me. I seldom see the Saints that they are not surrounded with a halo of light; they wear rich and precious armor, as it is reasonable they should. I see them always under the same forms, and have never found in their discourse any discrepancies. I know how to distinguish one from the other, and this as well by the sound of their voices as by their salutation. They come often without my calling upon them. But when they do not come, I pray to the Lord that He will send them to me, and never have I needed them but they have visited me."

These judges were nearly all ecclesiastics, selected by the Bishop of Beauvais for this particular work, sixty in all—bishops, writers of theology, mitred abbots, etc.; men skilled in all the subtleties of theological fence. She was a peasant girl, nineteen years of age, who could not even read and write. The only evidence that we have that they were not thoroughly depraved, is the fact that it was proposed to put her to the torture, and only three votes—from doctors of theology—were recorded in favor of this proposition. It is said, however, that the only reason why she was not tortured was the fact that being weak, she might die, and thus cheat the stake.

Of course she was found guilty. They found her to be: "A sorceress, a divinitress, an invoker of demons, a conjuress, superstitious, and entirely given to magic, thinking evil of the Catholic faith, sacrilegious, an idolatress, an apostate from the faith, a blasphemer of the name of God and of the Saints, scandalous, seditious, a disturber of the peace, exciting to war, cruel, wishing for the effusion of human blood, entirely abandoned and in variance with the sense of decency and shame, taking the dress of a man-at-arms as her habiliment, contemning and despising the law of God and of nature, and ecclesiastical discipline before God and men, a seducer of princes and peoples, consenting to the adoration of her person and allowing her hands and vestments to be kissed, to the great contempt and injury of the honor and the worship of God, therefore demanding that she be declared a heretic, and legitimately punished according to divine and canonical law."

She was sentenced to be burned alive, and this determination was kept concealed from her till the arrival of the day appointed for the execution. When told of it by her confessor, she exclaimed, in her misery, "Alas for me! It is dreadful that my healthy, youthful body, all unspotted, must this day be destroyed and reduced to ashes! Ah, it were better for me to be beheaded seven times over than to be burned to death!"

While on the scaffold, a sermon was preached to her from the text, "When one member suffers, all the other members suffer also." The discourse concluded with the words, "Depart in peace, the Church can no longer protect thee."

Then the Bishop of Beauvais, her relentless persecutor, who

had wielded the mighty ecclesiastical power against her, read the sentence:—

"In the name of God, Amen. We, thy lawful judges, found thee, Jeanne, called the Pucelle, guilty of apostacy, of idolatry, of invoking the devil, and of various other crimes; but as the Church ever opens its arms to receive the penitent, so we, believing that thou didst truly abjure and swear never to relapse into thy delusions, admitted thee again to repentance, as one resolved evermore to dwell in the unity of the Church. But thy heart was led astray by the Prince of lies, and thou art fallen back into thy errors, even as a dog returns to its vomit. Thou didst abjure thy errors with a false heart and not in good faith, as thou hast thyself acknowledged. Therefore, by the present sentence, we proclaim thee a relapsed heretic, and a withered branch. And lest thou corrupt others, we cast thee out of the bosom of the Church, and we deliver thee over to the temporal authorities, praying them to deal mildly and humanely by thee, and to rest satisfied with the death of thy body and the destruction of thy members."

As Madden* says, from whom I quote this account: "This last phrase is merely the deceitful form proper to the ecclesiastical sentence of death, for the temporal judge was far more under subjection to the inquisition than to the temporal powers of France, and by the rights delegated to the Church was liable to be himself accounted heretical, if he did not consign the person thus given over to him to the flames." And then she was burnt to death, and her ashes thrown into the river.

* Phantasmata. London, 1857, p. 186.

It was, therefore, in thorough consistency that the Church, bearing in mind its former action, recently refused to canonize this high-minded and virtuous maid. Perhaps a hundred or two years from now it will act differently in regard to another ecstatic who is fortunate enough during her lifetime to receive the favor of those who have the management of such things, and to whose history during the last few years I ask the attention of the reader.

Bernadette Soubirous, according to the account given by M. Henri Lasserre *, whose book is prefaced by a letter of approval from his Holiness the Pope, a young girl of Lourdes, in the south of France, went out one day with her two sisters to gather dry wood on the neighboring hills. On their way they had to cross a brook, and they stopped at the bank to take off their *sabots*. Bernadette was behind the other two, and being the only one who had on stockings, she stooped to take them off. It was about noon, and the *Angelus* was about to sound from all the bells of the neighboring villages.

She was in the act of taking off her stockings when she heard a sound as if a wind was rushing by her. To her surprise the poplars which bordered the banks of the river were in a state of complete repose, there being not the slightest ruffle of the leaves.

"I am deceived," she said to herself.

And remembering still the rushing sound she had heard, she did not know what to think.

Again she began to take off her stockings.

* Notre Dame de Lourdes, Paris, 1874.

And again the sound as if the wind were rushing by passed through her ears.

Bernadette raised her head, looked in front of her and uttered a loud cry, or rather, as M. Lasserre says, she would have uttered a loud cry if she had not been choked with fear. She trembled in all her limbs, and fell to the earth dazzled, completely overcome by what she had seen; she crouched on the ground on both knees and waited in terror for what was to come. For in a niche formed by nature, in the rock, stood a female figure of incomparable splendor. There was nothing fantastical or vague about this lovely being. She appeared to be a real woman, and the light that came from the aureola above her head, and from her whole body, though of surpassing brightness, did not hurt the eyes.

She was of middle height; she seemed to be quite young, and she had all the grace of a girl of twenty; but without detracting in the least from the delicacy and beauty of her form, there was at the same time, an air of eternal grandeur about it, which was in entire accordance with the fitness of things. Her face was oval, her eyes blue, her lips bore an expression of divine gentleness and love, her forehead appeared to express supreme wisdom—that is to say, the knowledge of all things, united to a virtue without limits.

The garments worn by this heavenly being were of an unknown material, and were doubtless, as M. Lasserre says, manufactured in a mysterious workshop, where lilies of the valley are made into textile fabrics; for they were as white as the immaculate snows of the mountains, and more magnificent in their simplicity than the gorgeous vestments worn by Solomon, when arrayed in all his glory. Her robe long and *er. train*, fell in chaste folds, allowing her feet to be seen as they stood upon the rock, pressing lightly a branch of eglantine. On each one of her feet, which were in a state of original nudity, bloomed the mystical golden colored rose.

In front a girdle, blue as the heavens, and tied half around the body, fell in two long bands which almost touched her feet. Behind, enveloping in its fulness her shoulders, and the upper part of her arms, was a white veil, which was fastened to her head and reached to the lower border of her robe.

There were neither rings, nor necklace, nor diadem, nor jewels; none of the ornaments with which human vanity, from all time, has loved to ornament her. A chaplet, of which the beads were as white as drops of milk, and of which the chain was as yellow as the harvest corn, fell from her hands, fervently clasped as they were. The beads of the chaplet glided one after the other through her fingers. Sometimes the lips of this Queen of Virgins were still. Instead of reciting her rosary she was then perhaps listening to the eternal echo in her heart of the angelic salutation, and to the murmur of the invocations coming from the earth. Each bead as she touched it was doubtless a shower of celestial graces, falling on souls as the drops of dew fall upon flowers.

She was silent, but afterwards her own words, and the miraculous facts mentioned, attested that she was really the immaculate Virgin, the very august and very holy Mary, the Mother of God.

It must be admitted that, considering the state of mental confusion into which Bernadette was thrown by this sudden appearance, she had a wonderful perception for the details of face, form, and dress, of the celestial figure before her. She tried to make the sign of the cross, but her agitation was so great that she could not raise her arm from her side. But the figure, as if to encourage her, made the sign with infinite grace, and then Bernadette, partially nerving herself, ran over her rosary, and as she finished it, the apparition disappeared and she was left alone.

No one believed the account she gave, even her mother regarding it as based on hallucination; but she saw the figure again, though her companions, not being gifted with the power of seeing spiritual things, saw only Bernadette fall on her knees, her face illumed with the light of ecstasy, as she gazed towards the place where she declared she perceived the Virgin. On another occasion two women went with her to the grotto, but though Bernadette saw the Virgin and fell on her knees at the sight, her two companions, as the others, saw only Bernadette, whose countenance was again transfigured by ecstasy.

After that, Bernadette was told by the Virgin that she wanted a church built on the spot. The water of the spring in the grotto became suddenly possessed of healing powers, and though the government attempted for a time to put a stop to the spread of the belief in Bernadette's visions, it was found to be impossible to do so, especially after a commission appointed by the bishop had rendered a report in favor of their authenticity. The rest is well known; the church was built by the contributions of the pilgrims who visited the place, either for purposes of devotion or to bathe in the healing pool, and the water of Lourdes became famous for the wonderful cures it accomplished. It is now exported to all parts of the world, and even in the city of New York is in extensive use as a therapeutical agent, its qualities being miraculous, according to the belief of those who place faith in its virtues.

This is the same old story over again, simply clothed in a new dress—a story that in one form or another has been repeated a thousand times, and that is probably destined to be reiterated again and again, while the world lasts, and the human mind continues to be constituted as it now is. But we, who know how to take such recitals at their true value, can derive from them many a lesson of use to us, in our dealings with men and women of sound and unsound minds and bodies. That thousands have been cured by the water of Lourdes admits of no doubt. Such facts are, however, only another group to be added to those embracing the results of the royal touch, the powder of sympathy, the metallic tractors, mesmerism, the acts of the Zouave Jacob and of Dr. Newton, and the bread pills and colored water, which, when taken in faith, are fully as miraculous in their effects as the water of Lourdes. And again, we see how prone man is to view facts "unequally," as Czermak puts it; to accept the most improbable explanation that can be offered of matters with which he is not wholly familiar, and while wise, as a child of the world ordinarily is in the conduct of his worldly affairs, a very prince of fools when an appeal is made to his sense of the marvellous.

There are few books of its kind more instructive, if read with a mind free from superstition and full of the knowledge of the wonderful workings of the human intellect, than the "*Notre Dame de Lourdes*" of M. Lasserre, and no one can rise from its perusal without being impressed with a sense of the incomparable adaptability of the Roman Catholic Church to the wants of those who are guided more by emotion than by reason, more by faith than by facts; and these constitute the majority of the human race.

As to Bernadette, let the reader recall to mind the circumstances under which she first saw the vision. She was stooping down in the act of taking off her stockings. The position was one which was calculated to accelerate the flow of blood to her brain, and to retard its return. A temporary cerebral congestion was thus induced, a condition particularly favorable to the production of hallucinations, as has already been pointed out. The roaring sound in the ears when there was no wind, was also the result of the augmented quantity of blood in the cerebral vessels.

Then, M. Lasserre repeatedly speaks of her ecstatic condition. "Suddenly Bernadette's countenance appeared to be transfigured, and it was in reality transfigured. An extraordinary emotion was depicted on her face, and her beaming expression seemed to be the result of a divine light."* "They (her two companions,) perceived that the features of the child were transfigured by ecstasy."† "Bernadette, ravished in ecstasy, gazed upon the immaculate beauty before her."‡ And again: "A minute afterwards her forehead appeared to become illuminated and radiant. The blood did not appear to rush to her face; on the contrary, she looked somewhat paler than natural, as if nature receded a little in the presence of the apparition which was before her. All her features seemed to

* Op. cit., p. 37. † Id., p. 41. ‡ Id., p. 42.

be enlarged, and as if in a higher sphere, in a country of glory, to express feelings and things which do not belong to this world. Her mouth, half open, was expressive of the admiration which filled her soul, and which appeared to raise her towards heaven. Her eyes, fixed and beaming with happiness, gazed on the beauty invisible to others, but which all felt to be present, which all, thus to speak, saw reflected in the face of the child. This poor little peasant girl, so ordinary in her natural state, seemed now not to belong to this earth.

All those who have seen Bernadette in ecstasy, speak of the spectacle as a thing quite without analogy in the world."*

So much for the orthodox account. The fact of ecstasy is admitted, but it is contended that while in this state the girl saw the Virgin Mary, although no one else, of the hundreds who went with her to the grotto, saw anything at all but the girl herself in the ecstatic state. If this kind of thing can be true, facts go for nothing. I have had under my own immediate charge fifty girls and women, who, in the condition of ecstasy, have had visions of, from God himself, down to the school-mistress who had locked them up in dark closets. That there were many sensible people who held this view in regard to Bernadette is very evident from M. Lasserre's admissions. Thus the editor of the "*Lavedan*," in detailing the events in question, said:

"Three children of early ages had gone out to collect the branches, which had been cut from some trees near the town. The girls were surprised by the proprietor of the

* Op. cit., p. 63.

land, and fled as fast as their legs could carry them to one of the grottos near the road through the forest of Lourdes. We shall not stop to detail the thousand versions which have been given of this occurrence; we will only say that the young girl, with a wax taper in her hand, and escorted by more than five hundred people, goes every morning to pray at the entrance of the grotto. There she is seen to pass from a state of profound and sighing meditation into a most pronounced condition of ecstasy. Tears flow from her fixed eyes, which remain constantly turned towards that part of the cave where she believes she sees the figure of the Blessed Virgin. Everything leads us to suppose that the poor visionary is the subject of catalepsy."

Of such people as the editor of the "*Lavedan*" M. Lasserre speaks with becoming disdain.

"Some physicians," he says, "some autocthonous Socrates, some local philosophers, calling themselves Voltairians to make us believe they have read Voltaire, bristling up against their curiosity, held it to be a point of honor not to visit the grotto with the stupid crowd, which daily grew in size. This is what almost always happens; the fanatics of "Free Examination" holding the principle of only examining what suits them. For them no fact is worthy of attention which is capable of overturning the inflexible dogmas they have learned in the *Credo* of their journal. From the height of their infallible wisdom, on the steps of their shops, on the terrace in front of the cafés, from the windows of the club houses, these spirits of the first order saw, with supreme disdain, the innumerable human souls which sauntered along on their way to the grotto."

These "disdainful spirits" were probably silenced, if not

convinced. Some of these days perhaps they, or their descendants, will have more voice in restraining the delusional vagaries of their fellow-creatures than they seem to have had in the matter of Our Lady of Lourdes.

After the first paroxysm, it was no difficult matter for Bernadette to have others. The mere fact of her fixing her gaze steadily in one direction would have been sufficient to produce them, just as the similar paroxysms of hypnotism are caused in the human species, and even in animals. This fact is well-known to the people of many nations. Thus, in India the seeker for wisdom, the anchorite, is told to go to some place of solitude, to seat himself neither too high nor too low, to keep the head, neck and body immovable, to look fixedly at the point of his nose, and to remain calm, chaste, free from fear, and to think only of God. A similar method is followed in China.

The monks of Mount Athos enter into ecstasy by placing their thoughts on God and their eyes on the navel. Simeon Abbot, of the monastery of Xerocos, writes the following instructions: "Being in thy cell, shut the door, and seat thyself in a corner of the room. Turn thy thoughts and thy eyes towards the middle of thy belly, that is to say, to thy navel. Hold thy breath, not even breathing through thy nose."

3. *Hystero-Epilepsy.* The combination of hysteria with epilepsy has long been recognized as one of the most frightful affections to be found in the whole range of neurological medicine. It is the condition which more frequently than any other led to the idea in former times—an idea which, however, as I shall presently show, holds its own among theologians of the present day—that demons entered the body and produced the

symptoms of the disorder by tearing and contorting it for diversional or malicious purposes.

An attack of hystero-epilepsy is characterized by the occurrence of convulsions more or less resembling those of epilepsy. There is usually, in the first place, a spasm resembling such as characterizes tetanus or lock jaw, as it is popularly called. During this stage the body is bent backward so as to resemble a bow in shape. Then follow convulsions, during which the body is violently agitated; there is frothing at the mouth, the urine is sometimes passed involuntarily and occasionally the tongue is bitten. During all this period the patient is unconscious.

Next ensues a remarkable series of movements, at the beginning of which, or during their continuance, the patient recovers consciousness to such an extent as to answer questions, though there is not often recollection of the incidents that may have occurred. These movements are apparently voluntary, and consist of the most extraordinary contortions of the face, neck, trunk and extremities, so that superstitious or ignorant people would be very apt to imagine the existence of an internal or external diabolical agency. During the continuance of this part of the paroxysm, the patient tears with the hands and teeth anything tearable that comes within reach, and continually utters inarticulate sounds or words, apparently in relation with the ideas passing through the mind. Finally the purely hysterical element ceases to predominate, and the patient alternately weeps and laughs, and gradually acquires a knowledge of what is passing around.

During the whole of the paroxysm the face is flushed, the

pupils are moderately contracted, the pulse is accelerated, the perspiration is increased in quantity, and the respiration is hurried and irregular.

But there are numerous deviations from this type. Sometimes the tetanic spasm is wanting, and again it, or some modification of it, may constitute the most marked part of the convulsive period. Thus in a lady who was lately under my charge the paroxysm began with the bending of the body, and the bowlike form was at once relaxed, and again assumed to be again relaxed, and so on for over half an hour, during which time the patient was sobbing, groaning, and shrieking alternately.

In a case now under my charge the patient, a woman, has daily attacks at about the same hour—three o'clock p. m.,—which are more distinctly tetaniform in the beginning than any that have come under my observation. They consist of a series of spasms, during the first part of which the body is extremely rigid. The convulsion is, however, unlike others that have come under my notice, very slowly developed. The body extended at full length in the recumbent position gradually becomes exceedingly rigid, the legs are slightly separated, the arms are pressed closely to the sides, the jaws are tightly closed and the gaze fixed. Respiration is entirely suspended and the heart beats rapidly, sometimes as frequently as one hundred and sixty pulsations in a minute. Then the body is slowly bowed so that the head and heels alone touch the bed, and is so rigid and strongly arched that no ordinary force, such as a powerful man can exert, suffices to overcome the extreme tonicity of the muscles. In about a minute from the beginning of the rigidity the spasm suddenly relaxes, and with a long-drawn inspiration the paroxysm ends to be again resumed in a few minutes with a like sequence. In the accompanying woodcut (Fig. 8) is an exact representation of this patient when the tetanic spasm is at its height.

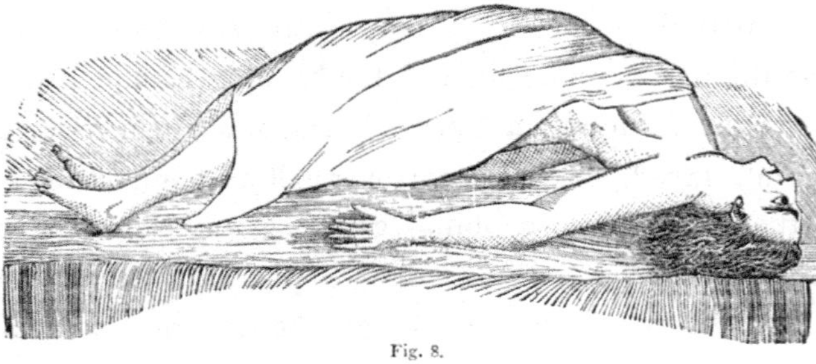

Fig. 8.

No one has written with greater effect in regard to the manifestations of hysteria and hystero-epilepsy than Charcot. As a most striking instance of this latter affection I cite from him the following instance,* already referred to in another communication under the head of ecstasy.

Ler., aged forty-eight, is a patient well known to all physicians who visit the Salpêtrière as one of the most remarkable instances extant of hystero-epilepsy. Her menstruation has ceased for four years, and yet all the neurotic symptoms persist. She is a demoniac, a possessed, and presents a striking example of that type of hysteria manifested by the "Jerkers" in "Methodist camp meetings," and who exhibit in their paroxysms the most frightful attitudes.

* "Leçons sur les Maladies du Système nerveux," Paris, 1872–73, p. 301, *et seq.*

The probable origin of these nervous phomonema in Ler. deserves to be noted. She has had, as she says, a series of frights. At eleven years of age she was terrified by a furious dog, at sixteen she was frightened at the sight of the corpse of an assassinated woman, and again about the same time when going through a wood by robbers, who attacked her and took away her money.

With her, there are various local manifestations of hysteria, consisting of anæsthesia of one half of the body, tenderness over the ovaries, semi-paralysis of various parts, and at times contractions of the limbs on the right or left side. The attacks are characterized at first by epileptiform and tetaniform convulsions, after which come extensive movements of an intentional character in which the patient assumes the most hideous postures, recalling the attitudes which history ascribes to demoniacal possessions. At the moment of the attack she is seized with delirium, which evidently turns on the facts which have produced the initial seizure. She hurls invectives at imaginary persons: "Scoundrels! robbers! brigands! Fire, fire! Oh the dogs, they bite me." When the convulsive part of the accession is over, there ensue generally, hallucinations of sight. She sees frightful animals, skeletons and spectres. Her power of swallowing food is impaired for several days, and the tongue is more or less contracted, leading to indistinctness of her articulation.

Later, M. Bourneville * has given an account of Ler. somewhat fuller than that of M. Charcot. In illustration of the period of contortions, I take from M. Bourneville's excellent

* Louise Lateau, ou la stigmatisée Belge. Paris, 1875, p. 38, et seq.

monograph the accompanying wood cut, (Fig. 9) made from a sketch taken on the spot, by Mr. Charcot.

A case at this time is under my care, in which phenomena very similar to those exhibited by Ler. are present. The patient is a girl who was brought to me after various remedies,

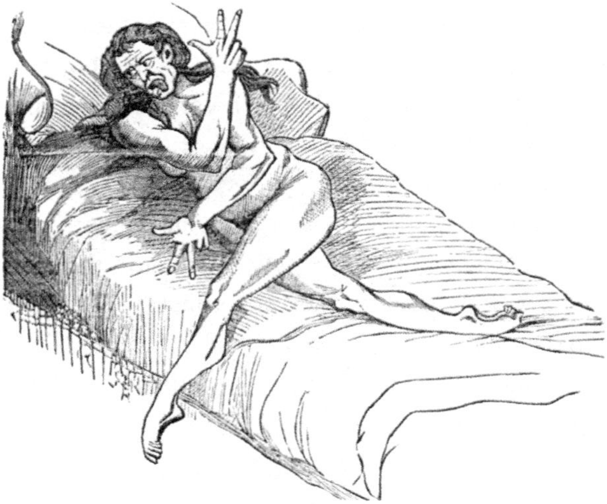

Fig. 9.

calculated to exorcise a supposed demon, had been employed. Although a Protestant, she had been taken to a "Christian Brother," who had laid his hands on her head, as her mother informed me, and had bid the devil depart, at the same time washing her with holy water. These means not succeeding, the water of Lourdes was next drunk and the forehead bathed with it. But these means also failed. Evidently Protestant devils are not amenable to Catholic spiritual therapeutics. She was then brought to me, and I had the opportunity of seeing her in a paroxysm.

It began with slight tetanic rigidity, then there were general clonic convulsions, epileptiform in character, with foaming at the mouth, and then the consciousness having been regained, the volitional muscular contractions made their appearance, as well as a higher state of delirium. The face twitched, the tongue was protruded, the eyes rolled. She seized books and other articles within her reach and hurled them about the room. She swore fearfully, and uttered the most obscene words with a horrible leer on her face. Then she threw herself on the floor and kicked, rolled and tossed about without regard to decency, or the safety of her own or others' limbs. She dashed her head against a chair, scratched her face, tore her hair, beat her breast, and almost entirely divested herself of clothing. Finally she fell asleep utterly exhausted, and did not awake for several hours. She was then sore from head to foot, and professed—evidently with truth—that she had no recollection of what had taken place. Such a case as this would, undoubtedly, at a not very remote anterior period have been regarded, almost without a dissentient voice, as one of diabolical or demoniacal possession, and even now there are not wanting learned and pious theologians, Catholic and Protestant, who would certainly thus designate it, for it fulfils in all respects the description given of such cases, both in ancient and modern times. Thus if we go back to the writers of the New Testament, we find the phenomena well described. There are convulsive movements, the body is contorted. the patient cries out, he foams at the mouth, falls down and then reposes.* The patient is torn, he foams at the mouth, gnashes his teeth.† He falls on the ground and wallows foaming.‡ He is contorted (vexed), falls sometimes into the fire and sometimes into the water.§

Delitzsch ‖ admits that these are the symptoms of epilepsy, but he very weakly attempts to make a distinction between the ordinary disease and that produced by the entrance of a devil into the human body, in that, *plus* these symptoms, one of the subjects was deaf and dumb. But it very often happens that patients are both epileptic and deaf and dumb, and that the cure of all the morbid conditions takes place at one time, being due as they are to an essential anatomical lesion, or some hysteroid state.

In contending for the reality of obsession and possession, Delitzsch, with a degree of learning and ability which it is lamentable to see wasted in such a cause, endeavors to locate the situation of the devil who has taken up his abode in the human organism. According to him the soul itself can never be invaded, and however strongly such a view may have been held, it must now be given up, as he says the locality of possession is the human body. "In this—and indeed just where the soul exerts an influence upon it by means of the nervous system, and receives reacting influence from it—the demon establishes himself, but from here outward exercises a forcible influence, extending itself to soul and spirit: to the soul at once so far as he makes the corporiety, *e. g.*, the instrument of speech, a means of his self-manifestation, and thereby dislodges the soul

* Luke ix. 39–42. † Mark viii. 18. ‡ Mark ix. 20. § Matt. xvii. 15.

‖ A System of Biblical Psychology. English Translation. Edinburgh, 1875, p. 348.

from its relation of power to the body that it vitalizes; to the spirit inasmuch as he degrades the will to a mere potentiality and places it in fetters that cannot be broken. So this affects the nature of man even to its very foundation. Even to the will, and thus even to the root of the soul and of the spirit, his influence penetrates. He binds the will in a magical manner, and makes it subservient to himself, and thus deprives the entire man of independence and of all further power over himself."*

Nor does the learned author stop here. He believes in the ability of man to form pacts or covenants with the devil—witchcraft. Thus he says:

"Nevertheless, that prevalence of demoniacal disorders, especially of possession, had also certainly a deep psychological reason in the superstition of that day, in virtue of which it was mingled with all kinds of magic. Superstition is not absolutely a mere subjective, guiltless delusion; and, moreover, it is not a complication which is dissolved by truly scientific illumination into a mere nothing. It opens the human soul to demoniacal influences just as much as faith does to divine. And witchcraft is not empty, guiltless legerdemain, and neither is it an empty fraud, disclosing itself to intelligent cultivation; it is, in its often sufficiently undeniable reality, the fearful opposite of the sacred miracles, which apart from God sets in movement created powers." †

Now what is the logical practical deduction from this? Obviously, that, if there are individuals capable of entering into contracts with demons or devils to torment their fellow beings, they ought to be put out of the world as rapidly as the machin-

* Op. cit., p. 355.

† Op. cit., p. 360.

ery of the law can be brought to bear against them. Burning at the stake would be a merited punishment for such fearfully degraded creatures. The error of our ancestors was not in the conclusions at which they arrived, but in the premises from which they reasoned. Admitting the truth of these, and they were perfectly right in consigning children and old men and women to the stake, the scaffold and the water. And Dr. Delitzsch, the Protestant professor of theology in the University of Leipsic, tells us they were right, and he says this in our day, right into our ears! Doubtless this very talented divine, who inveighs against superstition in the same breath with which he expresses his belief in witchcraft, would send Bernadette Soubirous to the category of fanatical and bigoted papists, and smile in derision at his Holiness the Pope, for writing approvingly to M. Lasserre and speaking kindly of Bernadette. But the Pope and his Church are at heart consistent, and it does seem to us—in our ignorance perhaps—that consistency is a virtue which those who set up to be teachers of mankind in the knowledge of eternal and never-changing truths, might cultivate with more advantage to themselves and their disciples. The Catholic Church believes in the possibility of possession, and it supplies a formula to its ministers by which demons are to be exorcised. This is the formula which exorcised the devils who had entered the body of the hystero-epileptic girl whose case I have just detailed: R. zinci bromidi ʒi; sodii bromidi, ℥i; aquæ, ℥iv; M. ft. sol. Sig. A teaspoonful in water three times a day. Demons of the present time have a great antipathy to the bromides, and in most cases they refuse to dwell in any body into which any one of the saints of that company obtains a lodgment.

CHAPTER XVI.

STIGMATIZATION.

IT is claimed by the Catholic Church (not, be it understood, as an article of faith which all must believe,) that there have been instances in which certain highly-favored individuals have, through miraculous agency, been marked in a manner to represent the wounds which Christ received in the crucifixion. When fully developed, these wounds consist of one in the palm of each hand, one on the dorsum of each foot, each indicating the place where a nail was inserted in the act of nailing Jesus to the cross, and one in the side, which represents the thrust of the spear which the Roman soldier is reported to have made. In some cases there have been, in addition, signs upon the forehead, which stand for the lacerations produced by the crown of thorns; and others in various parts of the body, which are interpreted according to the fancy of the subject. To some of these remarkable instances of the consequences of religious fervor I propose to ask the attention of the reader before entering into the consideration of the philosophy of the occurrences.

Görres * admits that in all the periods of Christian antiquity

* Op. cit., t. ii., p. 202.

there is not to be found a single example of stigmatization, properly so-called. The first to exhibit this mark of divine favor was St. Francis of Assisium, who was born in 1186, who died October 4th, 1226, and who, in 1224, became marked in the manner mentioned. In memory of the event a special day, the 17th of September, in every year was set apart as a feast of the Holy Stigmata by Pope Benedict XI.

One morning—the day of the exaltation of the cross—as St. Francis was praying on the mountain-side, he experienced a violent desire to be crucified with Christ. At the same time he saw a seraph descend from heaven towards him. This celestial being had six fiery and luminous wings, and as he approached, St. Francis saw between the wings, the figure of a man crucified, his arms and legs extended. Two of the wings were elevated above his head, two were used in flying, and the other two covered the body. Filled with astonishment at this sight, he nevertheless felt great joy that God had thus favored him, and at the same time profound grief at the painful spectacle of which he was a witness, and which pierced his heart like a sword. When the apparition had faded from his sight, there remained in his soul the most fervent emotions, and on his body very marvellous impressions, for on each hand and each foot was the mark of a nail, and in the right side a wound, such as would have been made with the point of a spear. These wounds were large, and blood flowed from them. In the middle of those in the hands and feet were nails like nails of iron. They were black, hard, with a head above and a point below, but though movable to some extent they could not be withdrawn. St. Clara tried to pull them out after St. Francis was dead, but was unable to do so. After receiving these wounds he could move his fingers and use his hands and feet as before. Nevertheless, walking was difficult to him, and therefore in his journeys he usually went on horseback. The wound of the side was deep and of the width of three fingers, as one of the brothers, who had by chance touched it, testified. His clothing was often stained with the blood which flowed from it.

There was never formed in his wounds any appearance of gangrene, nor even of suppuration; and the saint never employed any remedy for the purpose of curing them. It was regarded as miraculous, that notwithstanding his sufferings and the continued loss of blood, he lived for two years after receiving the stigmata.

The history of Christine de Stumbele is one of the most remarkable that has come down to us. She was born in 1242 at Stumbele, a village situated a few miles from Cologne. When she was only six years old the Lord appeared to her under the form of a beautiful young man, and said to her, "My dear daughter, I am the Lord Jesus; give thyself entirely to me, and continue always in my service." At nine years of age she went to live with the sisters at Cologne. There she led a life of prayer, austerities and ecstasies. At fifteen years began the diabolical temptations to which fuller reference will presently be made, and which lasted for thirty-one years. These were considered by the sisters to be epileptic, and they sent Christine home to her parents. These attacks prevented her being admitted to the sisterhood at Stumbele.

Christine had remained with her parents ten years, continually subject to these diabolical assaults, when she was visited by Pierre de Dacie, who had prayed to God to show him a true saint, and who sent him to Christine. Hardly had Pierre entered her house when she was seized by an invisible hand and thrown violently against the wall, with such violence that the house shook. Although this was repeated seven times, Christine exhibited neither impatience nor pain. Pierre, touched with compassion, placed a mattrass against the wall, so as to soften the violence of the blows in case of fresh assaults. But she soon began to groan with pain on account of wounds, which she said she had received in her feet. On examination, a fresh wound was found on each foot, from which blood flowed. This was repeated several times. Afterwards, while she was talking with Pierre, she again began to groan, and on his asking what was the matter, she replied, "I am wounded in the knee." After a few moments she passed her hand under her robe and drew out a nail, which she showed him, and which he declared had a most extraordinary degree of heat, as if in fact it were newly arrived from hell. Towards midnight he joined his companion monk, and began the recital of the office, but had barely got to "Laudes," when they heard such a noise in Christine's room that they were obliged to interrupt their prayers and go to her relief. The young girl suffered horribly, and appeared to be dying. A moment afterwards she drew from under her clothing another nail, red-hot, and of hideous shape; and putting it in the hand of his companion (after it had cooled, it is to be hoped), said, "See what has been wounding me!" The two monks looked at this horrible nail, and were struck with stupor and fear. Pierre requested permission to keep it as a souvenir; "and," he says, in his account of the matter, "I have kept it to this day." In the morning, the two brothers departed on their way to Cologne, and Pierre thanked God for having allowed him to witness all these manifestations.

The foregoing details in regard to St. Christine de Stumbele are taken almost literally from the recent work of Dr. Imbert-Gourbeyre,* professor in the school of medicine of Clermont Ferrand, in Belgium, who quotes the principal part from Pierre de Dacie, with full acceptance of all that is stated. It is lamentable that a member of a profession, so little prone to be deceived in matters of the kind, should exhibit such ignorance of his own science, and such credulity and superstition. We shall see hereafter that he is not the only Belgian physician who views facts "unequally."

But to continue the account of Christine—

Pierre made a second visit to Stumbele, and was invited to dine with the curé in company with Christine. After the repast, one of those present undertook to chant "*Jesu dulcis memoria*," but he had hardly begun before Christine was taken with ecstasy, was motionless, rigid in all her limbs and completely insensible. She could not even be seen to breathe. "I wept with joy," says Pierre, "stupefied with this miracle, and I thank God for granting me such a favor. I could not attribute it either to nature or to man, and I venerated the divine presence."

Christine remained in this condition for several hours, stretched out on a bench, her body wrapped in her veil. Then she began to cry and sob, and her body became agitated. Her

* Les Stigmatisées. Louise Lateau, etc., 2d édition. Paris, 1873, t. i, p. 268.

breath then began to return, though at first, very feebly. Finally she began to murmur a few words, such as "O my well-beloved! O my spouse!" and then she went into such a state of jubilation that her body trembled with excess of emotion.

On another occasion while in a profound state of ecstasy, her body exhaled a most delicious perfume, "the odor of sanctity," which has been exhibited by many other holy persons. It must be confessed, however, that if the stories which have come down to us, relative to the personal habits of most of the holy men and women whose histories have been written, are true, the odor exhaled from their bodies could not have been of a very delectable character.

Christine had numerous temporary stigmatizations, which always took place on Good Fridays and lasted a few days. The first one occurred in 1267—being preceded by the crown of thorns, which came on Tuesday of Passion Week, and by the bloody sweat which occurred on Holy Thursday. The following morning she had the five wounds.

Pierre has left a description of the stigmata as he observed them on one occasion. There was a wound in the palm of each hand of about the size of a shilling piece. The flesh was exposed but the abrasion was only superficial. The stigmata on the backs of the hands were in complete relation, both as regarded size and situation, with those on the palms. All these wounds remained but for eight days, diminishing little by little.

Subsequently the devil again began to torment her and her friends. Pierre, accompanied by another monk, paid her a visit, at the request of her father. They had saluted the young girl and had gone into the next room to dry their garments, when another clerical visitor who had taken a seat in front of the fire, was suddenly struck violently on his legs by an invisible hand, and at the same time covered with human excrement.

In a few minutes afterwards this was repeated. "I ascertained," said Pierre, "that the demon more than twenty different times during that night, covered Christine with excrement. Sometimes it was on her clothing, sometimes on her body, and on one occasion, though her head was veiled, it was covered with excrement as if with a paste. It was in her eyes, in her mouth, and it stuck so fast that it was difficult to remove it. "I must avow," continues Pierre, with great *naiveté*, "that some of it got on my hands."

These are filthy matters to talk or write about, and nothing but the necessity which I think exists for giving a true idea of the vagaries which hysterical women at times indulge in, causes me to place them before the reader. All of these phenomena —the sticking of sharp instruments into the body, the introduction of them into the various passages, the drinking of wine, and tricks with excrementitious substances, both of man and the lower animals, together with many others, which do not seem to have occurred to Christine de Stumbele, are common enough as manifestations of hysterical, or hysteroid affections.

But to return to the performances of this saintly creature.

The next night all the doings of the previous night were re-enacted with additions. "Towards the hour of midnight," he continues in his journal, "I asked Christine if she saw the demon. As for us, it was easy to know the presence of the demon by his acts—by all our senses, by the eyes, by the nose, by the touch, and even by the ears. Christine declared that she saw him all the time, even with her eyes closed, or covered with a veil. He took all possible forms. At that moment she only saw his figure, but it was hideous. However deformed it might be, it was always a human figure, having two great horns." Pierre asked whether or not the demon would go, if he sprinkled the chamber with holy water, and Christine replied that he would, but that he would soon return.

"The following day," says Dr. Imbert-Gourbeyre, * in his book published only three years ago, and prefaced with a letter of endorsement and approval from the Bishop of Nantes, "was passed tranquilly as was also the night, but on the third night the same scenes recommenced. Brother Wipert was then absolutely determined to recite the prayers of exorcism, in order to put the devil to flight. Christine, however, took occasion to say that it would be useless, and that she was still condemned to submit to the assaults of the devil, so long as the good God should determine. But Brother Wipert was obstinate and began to recite the formula. Hardly had he begun, however, when a tremendous noise was heard in the room, the candle was extinguished, and Brother Wipert panic-stricken, rose up and attempted to seek safety in flight. At that moment he felt a blow, and was covered with excrement. He rushed from the room repeating "O my God, I have lost an eye!" In the next chamber, before the fire and with hot water, he busied himself in washing his clothing, soiled by the demoniacal operation. The sisters helped him in his cleansing processes. Brother

* Op. cit., p. 285.

Wipert had been very badly treated. One-half of his body from head to foot was covered with liquid excrement. A few minutes afterwards, well cleaned, he entered Christine's room laughing. 'The devil,' said he, "has dirtied me all over and has given me such a blow that I thought at first he had put out my eye,' Pierre de Dacie could not help laughing also."

How it is possible for any person claiming to have a human brain normally constituted—that noblest work of God—to believe such stuff as this, passes comprehension.

It is scarcely worth while to inquire further into the acts of this filthiest of hysterical women, this most degraded of all the individuals who have pretended to stigmatization as the act of God. I will only further state, that her performances are contained in not less than one hundred and fifty folio pages in the collection of the Bollandists, extending over a period of twenty years, from 1267 to 1287, and that they are accepted as veritable acts of the devil and of God, according as one or the other was for the time being in the ascendency, by bishops, priests, deacons, and laity of the most important of all the Christian churches.

Yes, there is one thing more to state in regard to this woman who is honored as a saint, by the church that has recently refused canonization to Joan of Arc. Her relics were first taken to Niedeck, then, towards the end of the sixteenth century, to Juliers. Here in the year 1685, they were visited by Father Steinfunder, who reported that a green crown, the width of the finger, was in process of growing from the forehead to the occiput. When he saw it, it had reached the ears.

"God thus wished," said he, "to crown the chastity and the invincible patience of the virgin." In 1692 he inspected the relics a second time. The virginal crown was still growing, and it was sprinkled with red drops, which were symbolical of the points of insertion of the crown of thorns she had received during her life.

Veronica Giuliani had frequent ecstasies, during which she saw and conversed with Christ and the Virgin Mary. In one ot these interviews she prayed that she might be crucified with her Saviour, and the promise was given her that she should receive the stigmata on the following Good Friday. When that day arrived she had repeated ecstasies, and received the stigmata during one of her prayers. She saw the Lord attached to the cross, and His mother seated at His feet. She prayed to the Holy Virgin to intercede for her, knowing that of herself she could do nothing. The Holy Virgin promised to grant her prayer, and she immediately received an assurance from the Lord that He would cause her to remember Him in everything. Three times He asked her what she desired, and three times she answered that it was her wish to be crucified with Him. "I accord it to thee," said He, "but I wish you to be always faithful to me and I will give the grace thou needest by means of these wounds, which I now impress upon thy body as a sign of the gift I have bestowed upon thee." Immediately five brilliant rays emanated from the five wounds of the Saviour, and were directed towards her. In these rays she saw little flames. Four of them represented the nails and the fifth the lance. The nails and the lance seemed to be of gold, but were blazing at the same time. "The heart, the hands, and the feet of the

Saint were pierced. She experienced great pain, but simultaneously she felt herself transformed into Our Lord." *

Awakened from her ecstasy, she perceived that her arms were extended and rigid. She tried to look at the wound in her side, but she could not on account of the pain she felt in her hands; nevertheless, after renewed efforts, she succeeded, and then she saw that it was open, and that water and blood were pouring from it.

Doubts in regard to the truth of her story arose, and she was ordered by her confessor to submit to a very severe examination, which the inquisition ordered the bishop of her diocese to make in order to ascertain whether she was deceiving or not. This, according to Görres and other authorities, was of such a character that if she had been a fraud the fact would inevitably have been discovered. But she came triumphantly out of all her trials, and the stigmata were accepted as genuine gifts of God, according to the account she had given. Veronica was beatified by Pope Pius VII., and canonized by Gregory XVI., May 26th, 1839.

Dr. Imbert-Gourbeyre † gives a list of one hundred and forty-five persons who have received the stigmata, besides eight now living, known to him. He has reason to think there are many others now on the earth. America has only had one, and, according to Dr. Imbert-Gourbeyre, she is still living. In regard to her he gives the following details without, however, citing his authority. I quote them for what they may be worth:

" Vitaline Gagnon was born twenty years ago, of poor pa-

* Görres.—Op. cit. t. ii. p. 216.

† Les Stigmatisées. Palma D'Oria, etc., 2d edition. Paris, 1873, p. 263

rents, in the diocese of Quebec. From her earliest infancy she gave evidences of piety, and while quite a child experienced great delight in visiting the cemeteries and saying *Ave Marias* among the tombs. Hence she acquired a great regard for the souls in purgatory, who often rendered themselves visible to her to ask the benefit of her prayers. About the age of thirteen she entered the noviciate of the *Sœurs Hospitaliers* of Quebec, but she was obliged to leave by direction of her physicians, who declared that a cloistered life was not to be endured by one of her weak constitution. Some time afterwards she presented herself to the *Sœurs Grises* at Ottara [Ottawa ?], after being cured of a cough which was thought to be incurable. Threatened with being sent away on account of this cough, she prostrated herself at the feet of the Holy Virgin and coughed no more. She made her profession two years afterwards, and on the same day received the stigmata. Since that time the stigmata bleed, every Friday, and every time that she offers her sufferings with the object of obtaining a grace for any one who is commended to her prayers. Since her profession, now two years, she has taken no nourishment, and she suffers terribly. A little wine is all that has passed her lips. She has exteriorly all the signs of perfect health ; she is even stout. The water which flows from her wounds is always perfumed, and a person has only to remain in her room a few minutes to be quite impregnated with perfumes. She offers all her sufferings for the souls in purgatory. The author of this note states that he reports only what he knows and has seen."

Of the seven other stigmated individuals of the present day, I propose to consider at some length the main points in the histories of two, Palma d'Oria and Louise Lateau, and in so doing I shall avail myself of the works of those, who are firm believers in the miraculous interposition of God to produce the effects, of which they are said to be the subjects. These cases are very little known in this country. Instances of the kind are extremely rare among practical common sense nations, like those inhabiting the British Isles, and their descendants in America. Of the whole one hundred and fifty-three cases recorded by Dr. Imbert-Gourbeyre, but one—Jane Gray—was British, and hers is the most doubtful case in the list, for the fact rests only on the testimony of one Thomas Bourchier, an English minor brother, who asserts that she had the stigmata in the feet. Of the remainder, the very large majority are of Italy, and as Dr. Imbert-Gourbeyre says:

"Quel pays fut jamais si fertile en miracles?" *

To the account of a visit made to Oria for the purpose of studying the phenomena exhibited by Palma, made by Dr. Imbert-Gourbeyre, I am indebted for the following details:

Palma, at the time of the visit in 1871, was sixty-six years old, hump-backed, thin, small, and with light, expressive eyes. For several years she had not left the house, and was, on account of her sufferings, scarcely able to walk. Occasionally, when she felt particularly well, she took a few steps about the room supported by a cane. In her youth she had been very strong and active.

At the first interview, after some conversation in the course of which Palma declared that she had often seen Louise Lateau while in ecstasy, the doctor directed the conversation

* Op. cit., t. ii.

towards the subject of hallucination. While thus engaged and seated close to Palma, he felt her strike him gently on the arm, and at the same time saw the abbé, who had come with him, fall on his knees. He turned toward Palma; her eyes were closed, her hands clasped, her mouth wide open, and on her tongue he saw the host—the body of Christ. Immediately he fell on his knees also, and worshipped it. Palma protruded her tongue still farther, as if she wanted to give him every opportunity of seeing that the host was really there; then she ate it, closed her mouth and remained perfectly quiet on the sofa upon which she was reclining. It was then almost four o'clock in the afternoon, the day was fading, the room was badly lit by a little window, high from the floor. The miraculous host appeared to him to be as white as wax, and somewhat thick. On account of the little light, and the short time that this extraordinary communion lasted, he was unable to determine whether or not it was marked according to the custom of the church.

In regard to this wonderful event—that is, if it be not a fact viewed unequally—it is further to be said that Palma disclosed to Dr. Imbert-Gourbeyre, that two or three times, the holy element, which be it remembered is believed by the great majority of Christians to be the real body of Christ, was brought to her by the devil, and that then she refused it. Sometimes he had the figure of an angel, but she knew him by the sign of reprobation which he wore on his forehead—a little horn. Moreover she saw that the wicked creature hesitated, and was a little embarrassed. She intoned the *Gloria Patri*, and made the sign of the cross, and he instantly took flight and disappeared. In order to ascertain what it all meant, her confessor forbade her to receive the miraculous communion for eight days. Hardly had that period expired when Jesus Christ himself brought her the communion. Before giving it to her he made her recite the *Gloria Patri* three times. Then he said to her, "Have I fled as the demon did? No. Therefore reassure yourself. It is really I."

These miraculous circumstances had been going on for about two years when Dr. Imbert-Gourbeyre made his visit to Palma. Sometimes it was brought to her by Christ, as in the instance specified, or by some saint, as St. Peter, St. Vincent de Paul, St. Francis d'Assisi, in the company of her guardian angel, and other saints and angels. At other times it was brought by priests and confessors of the olden time, long since dead.

An Italian bishop stated, that at the moment of the miraculous sacrament on one occasion, he had seen the host flying through the air before entering Palma's mouth, but the doctor questioned her attendant on this point, and she declared that she had not seen that, and she assured him that the host was never seen by any one till it rested on Palma's tongue. The doctor inclines to the belief that the attendant was right, but he states that nevertheless a French apostolic missionary had asserted that he had seen the same thing.

Well, if the consecrated bread be really the body of Christ that was given for the salvation of the world, what horrible blasphemy to state such things of it, what vileness to believe them, what a barefaced imputation on the reason of man to spread these shocking details before him and ask him to accept them as true of the God he worships!

After witnessing the communion, Dr. Imbert-Gourbeyre was requested to withdraw into the adjoining room, while Palma got ready for her other performances. In a few minutes he was informed that all was in order. One of the women went in first and returning immediately, the others were invited to enter. The stigmatization had already begun on the forehead. He saw a stream of blood flowing from the left frontal eminence along the side of the nose. A handkerchief was given to Palma ; she held it to her nose for a moment and the hæmorrhage soon stopped. He examined the blood and found that it did not differ in appearance, color or temperature from ordinary blood. He then examined the handkerchief, and besides numerous rotund spots he perceived other figures resembling hearts, with stains of blood proceeding from them, indicating the flames of love. All this appeared to him to be very extraordinary, for though he had often seen people bleed from the nose, he had never seen them bleed like that.

After this incident Palma continued the performances—*actions de grace* he calls them—her hands clasped and her eyes closed. In the lower limbs, especially the left, there was a tremor like a nervous trembling which was soon quieted. After a few minutes she rubbed her hands together, made the sign of the cross and returned naturally to the conversation. He then examined her forehead and endeavored to ascertain where the blood had come from. The skin was intact without the least opening. She showed him above the right frontal eminence a hole in the cranium, from which at a former period, five little pieces of bone had been discharged. The opening was entirely covered over by the scalp, and he was surprised to find that there was no cicatrix. It was round, the end of his index finger entered it readily, and it was just such an opening as would have been produced by the crown of a trephine. At the time it was made, the skin opened to allow of the exit of the pieces of bone; then it closed without leaving the trace of a scar. It was the same with the stigmata. They closed at once without there being any marks to indicate the place whence the blood had flowed. This hole in the skull had been caused by some particular circumstances that no one was willing to reveal to him, but which he says are reported in the journal of the directors of this woman, and which will soon be published. Most medical men will come to the conclusion that it was due to caries and necrosis of the bone, of syphilitic origin.

During another visit Palma told Dr. Imbert-Gourbeyre that she had eaten nothing for seven years, but that she was obliged to drink frequently on account of the great internal heat, which like a fire consumed her. She then drank in his presence two carafes of water at one time, and the doctor states that "this water became so hot in her stomach that it was vomited boiling. She also had often ejected from her mouth oil, and another fluid of a balsamic character, in which, on standing for some time, bodies resembling the consecrated host were formed."

The doctor then relates the following details, which I give in his own words, in further illustration of the character of his mental organization and of the pretensions put forth by the woman, whose word seems to have been sufficient to convince him of anything at all, no matter how preposterous. Four years previously he had been so unfortunate as to lose by death his eldest child :

" A year after his death, I had met a woman of great renown for piety, and who was even regarded as a receiver of celestial communications. I had commended my poor Joseph to her. Some time after she assured me that my son was saved, and that he was in paradise. She declared that in a vision she had seen him near our Lord ; he was happy. Various circumstances, which it is useless to mention here, had caused me to believe in the truth of this asserted revelation. Being in Oria, I wished to have as much certainty as possible in regard to the matter, and as I knew that Palma was in spiritual communication with many pious souls scattered over the earth, I said to her in the course of our conversation, 'tell me, Palma, do you know M. —— de X——,' giving her the baptismal name of the woman in question. 'No sir,' she answered. " I then related to her my history in detail, taking care not to ask her opinion in advance, although I felt sure that she would explain the thing to me. She listened with the utmost attention to the superioress who translated my words, and when Mother Becaud came to say that the woman had had a vision of my son, and that he was in paradise, Palma stretched out her arm in a solemn manner as a sign of negative, and said to me, " 'He is saved, but he is still in purgatory.' "

'Is it possible ? Palma,' I cried, profoundly moved : 'Since you tell me this, you are in conscience bound to get him out of that place of expiation as soon as possible, and I commend him immediately to your prayers.'

" 'Yes, sir,' she said, 'I will pray for him, and when I am

sure of his deliverance, I will send you word by Father de Pace.

"The following morning at my visit I again commended my poor child to Palma, and on the following Friday evening on taking leave of her, I asked if she had prayed that morning for my son, 'No sir,' she answered. 'I will only do so on the day of All Saints.' 'Then' said I to Palma, 'will you allow madame the superioress to take the answer.' 'Very willingly said the seeress.' On the 7th of November, I received at Nice the following letter:

"Sir,

"'I have fulfilled the promise which I made to you in accordance with your wish to go to Palma on All Saints Day, in order to ascertain whether or not your wishes in regard to your son had been granted. That good soul assured me twice that he had gone to heaven that very morning, God be praised a thousand times!

"'Thus sir, I have done what I could for your consolation.

"'I have the honor to be, etc.

"'Sister Marie Becaud.'

"This letter was post marked at Oria, November 2d."

I should not venture to insult the intelligence of the reader with these idiotic details but for the reasons stated, and additionally, that they carry conviction with them to thousands of minds, honest doubtless, but which are accustomed to grovel in superstition, and falsehood, which they are unable to test by right standards.

A phase in Palma's spiritual pathology has been alluded to cursorily, but has not yet been considered with the fulness proper in connection with stigmatization, and that is the occurrence of hæmorrhagic spots on various parts of her body, and which she so managed as to convey the idea that they were symbolical of various holy things. On the back of her hand she convinced Dr. Imbert-Gourbeyre that she bled in the shape of the cross, and he gives a wood-cut representing a cross on the dorsum of the hand, a little above the space between the first and second fingers. This is surrounded by other rectilinear figures. On her breast and back, other figures were obtained by placing handkerchiefs on the parts. The doctor thus procured several mementoes of his visit, in the shape of pieces of linen stained with spots of blood somewhat resembling hearts, with flames coming out of them, suns, roses, crosses, etc. He gives several plates in his book representing these figures, of the reality of the miraculous formation of which he has not the slightest doubt.

Another phenomenon has also been mentioned incidentally, and that is the intense heat which Palma declared she felt, and which the doctor refers to as the "divine fire." He had brought with him from Paris, a thermometer to use in determining the extraordinary temperature of this fire. He examined her with this instrument while she felt this divine fire, but failed to find any abnormal increase; her pulse at the time was 72. "I made this experiment," he says, "to satisfy my scientific conscience, [God save the mark !] but I ought to say that I was ashamed of myself for presuming to measure this divine fire by such an instrument." He is right, science is not for him, or those like him.

On one occasion while Palma was in ecstasy, Antonietta,

who was near her, laid bare her chest a little, and cried with enthusiasm, "she is burning!" Dr. Imbert-Gourbeyre approached and smelt something like the burning of linen. The dress was opened and her chemise was found to be burnt on the left side just over the collar bone, and immediately below this, scorched in the shape of "a magnificent emblem representing a monstrance. The fire was invisible, but its traces were very evident."

In a note he states that it was affirmed that Palma's temperature on similar occasions had reached 100° centigrade, (212° Farenheit) a fact which he does not doubt, although his thermometer did not show it. "That her chemise," he says, "burnt by invisible fire, which escaped the thermometer, was more extraordinary than if the instrument had indicated a temperature of 100°."

I shall not stop now to comment further on the circumstances detailed by Dr. Imbert-Gourbeyre, and of which I have cited but a small part. I will only say at present that science and common sense would conclude in regard to Palma d'Oria,

1st. That she had probably at a former period contracted syphilis.

2d. That she was strongly hysterical.

3d. That she was the subject of purpura hæmorrhagica.

4th. That she was a most unmitigated humbug and liar.

And now we come to the consideration of a case of stigmatization which has greatly stirred both the theological and the scientific world of Europe—that of Louise Lateau—and here again I shall draw largely, though by no means exclusively, from the works of the believers in the miraculous production of the phenomena manifested.*

Louise Lateau was born at Bois-d'Haine, a small village in Belgium, on the 30th of January, 1850. She was reared in the utmost poverty, was chlorotic, and did not menstruate till she was eighteen years old. She loved solitude and silence, and when not engaged in work—and she does not appear to have labored much—she spent her time in meditation and prayer. She was subject to paroxysms of ecstasy, during which, as many other ecstasies, she spoke very edifying things, of charity, poverty, and the priesthood. She saw St. Ursula, St. Roch, St. Theresa, and the Holy Virgin. Persons who saw her in these states declared that, while lying on the bed, her whole body was raised up more than a foot high, the heels alone being in contact with the bed.

The stigmatization ensued very soon after these seizures. On a Friday she bled from the left side of her chest. On the

* For the theological view of this remarkable case the reader is referred to the following works, a part only of those written in support of her pretensions. "Louise Lateau de Bois-d'Haine, sa vie, ses extases, ses stigmates," etude Médicale, par le Dr. Lefebvre, Louvain 1873. "Les stigmatiseés Louise Lateau, etc.," par le Docteur A. Imbert-Gourbeyre Paris, 1873. "Biographie de Louise Lateau" par H. Van Looy, Tournai, Paris and Leipzig 1874. "Louise Lateau de Bois d'Haine etc." par le Dr. A. Rohling, Paris, 1874. "Louise Lateau, ihr Wunderleben u. s. w." Von Paul Majunke, Berlin, 1875.

Among the treatises in which the miracle is denied, and the phenomena attributed to either disease or fraud are ;" Louise Lateau ; Rapport Médicale sur la stigmatisée de Bois-d'Haine, fait a l'academie royale de médecine Belgique, par le Dr. Warlomont, Bruxelles and Paris, 1875. "Science et miracle, Louise Lateau, ou la stigmatisée Belge" par le Dr. Bourneville, Paris, 1875. "Les Miracles ;" par M. Virchow, Revue des cours scientifiques, January 23rd 1875.

following Friday this flow was renewed, and in addition, blood escaped from the dorsal surfaces of both feet ; and on the third Friday, not only did she bleed from the side and feet, but also from the dorsal and palmar surface of both hands. Every succeeding Friday the blood flowed from these places, and finally other points of exit were established on the forehead and between the shoulders.

At first these bleedings only took place at night, but after two or three months they occurred in the daytime, and were accompanied by paroxysms of ecstasy, during which she was insensible to all external impressions, and acted the passion of Jesus and the crucifixion.

M. Warlomont, being commissioned by the Royal Academy of Medicine of Belgium to examine Louise Lateau, went to her house, accompanied by several friends, and made a careful examination of her person. At that time, Friday morning at six o'clock, the blood was flowing freely from all the stigmata. In a few moments the sacrament would be brought to her, and then the second act of the drama would begin. The scene that followed can be best described in M. Warlomont's own words :

"It is a quarter-past six. 'Here comes the communion,' said M. Niels [a priest], 'kneel down.' Louise fell on her knees on the floor, closed her eyes and crossed her hands, on which the communion-cloth was extended. A priest, followed by several acolytes, entered ; the penitent put out her tongue, received the holy wafer, and then remained immovable in the attitude of prayer.

We observed her with more care than seemed to have been hitherto given to her at similar periods. Some thought that she was simply in a state of meditation, from which she would emerge in the course of half an hour or so. But it was a mistake. Having taken the communion, the penitent went into a special state. Her immobility was that of a statue, her eyes were closed ; on raising the eyelids the pupils were seen to be largely dilated, immovable, and apparently insensible to light. Strong pressure made upon the parts in the vicinity of the stigmata caused no sensation of pain, although a few moments before they were exquisitely tender. Pricking the skin gave no evidence of the slightest sensibility. A limb, on being raised, offered no resistance, and sank slowly back to its former position. Anæsthesia was complete, unless the cornea remained still impressionable. The pulse had fallen from 120 to 100 pulsations. At a given moment I raised one of the eyelids, and M. Verriest quickly touched the cornea. Louise at once seemed to recover herself from a sound sleep, arose and walked to a chair, upon which she seated herself. 'This time,' I said, 'we have wakened her.' 'No,' said M. Niels, looking at his watch, 'it was time for her to awake.'"

She remained conscious ; the blood still continued to flow ; the anæsthesia had ceased, her pulse rose to 120, and at the end of half an hour she was herself. "Our first visit ended here. At half-past eleven we made another. The poor child had resumed her attitude of extreme suffering, against which she contended with all the energy that remained to her. The wounds in the hands still continued to bleed. M. Verriest auscultated with care the lungs, heart, and great vessels, and found the *bruit de souffle*, which he had detected in the morning at the apex of the heart and over the carotids. The handle of a spoon pressed against the velum, the base of the tongue, and the pharynx, provoked no effort at vomiting. The glasses of our spectacles, as they came in contact with the air expired, were covered with vapor. As the patient appeared to suffer from our presence, we went away.

"We made our third visit at two o'clock. There were still fifteen minutes before the beginning of the ecstatic crisis, which always took place punctually at a quarter past two and ended at about half past four. The pupils at this time were slightly contracted, the eyelids were almost entirely closed; the eyes, looking at nothing, were veiled from our view. We tried in vain to attract her attention; her mind was otherwise engaged, and her pains were evidently becoming more intense. At exactly a quarter past two her eyes became fixed in a direction above and to the right. The ecstacy had begun.

"The time had now come to introduce those who were prompted by curiosity. This could now be done without inconvenience, for the ecstatic, for the ensuing two hours, would be lost to the appreciation of what might be passing around her. The room crowded, could hold about ten persons, but enough were allowed to enter to make the total twenty-five. These placed themselves in two ranks, of which the front one kneeling, allowed the rear ones to see all that was going on All this was done under the direction M. le Curé, who took every pains to give us a good view of what was going to happen.

"Louise was seated on the edge of her chair; her body, inclined forward, seemed to wish to follow the direction of her eyes, which did not look, but were fixed on vacancy. Her eyes were opened to their fullest extent, of a dull, lustreless appearance, turned above and to the right, and of an absolute immobility. A few workings of the lids were now observed and became more frequent if the eyelids were touched. The pupils, largely dilated, showed very little sensibility to light, and all that remained of vision was shown by slight winking when the hand was suddenly brought close to the eyes. The whole face lacked expression. At certain moments, either spontaneously or as a consequence of divers provocations, a light smile, to which the muscles of the face generally did not contribute, wandered over her lips. Then the face resumed its primitive expression, and thus she remained for the half-hour which constituted the 'first station.'

"The 'second station' was that of genuflection. It had failed at one time, but had again appeared. The young girl fell on her knees, clasped her hands, and remained for about a quarter of an hour in the attitude of contemplation. Then she arose and again resumed her sitting posture.

"The 'third station' began at three o'clock. Louise inclined herself a little forward, raised her body slowly, and then extended herself at full length, face downward, on the floor. There was neither rigidity nor extreme precipitation; nothing in fact, calculated to produce injuries. The knees first supported her body, then it rested on these and the elbows, and finally her face was brought in actual close contact with the tiled floor. At first the head rested on the left arm, but very soon the patient made a quick and sudden movement, and the arms were extended from the body in the form of a cross. At the same time the feet were brought together so that the dorsum of the right was in contact with the sole of the left foot. This position did not vary for an hour and a half. When the end of the crisis approached, the arms were brought close to the sides of the body, then suddenly the poor girl rose to her knees, her face turns to the wall, her cheeks become colored, her eyes have regained their expression, her countenance expands, and the ecstasy is at an end."

Further particulars are given, and an apparatus was constructed and applied to Louise's hand and arm so as to prevent any external excitation of the hæmorrhage. It was apparently shown that there was no such interference, for the blood began to flow at the usual time on Friday.

In addition to the stigmata and the paroxysms of ecstasy, Louise declared that she did not sleep, had eaten or drank nothing for four years, had had no fecal evacuation for three years and a half, and that the urine was entirely suppressed.

M. Warlomont examined the blood and products of respiration chemically, and satisfied himself of their normal character, except that the former contained an excessive amount of white corpuscles.

When being closely interrogated, Louise admitted that, though she did not sleep, she had short periods of forgetfulness at night. On M. Warlomont suddenly opening a cupboard in her room, he found it to contain fruit and bread, and her chamber communicated directly with a yard at the back of the house. It was therefore perfectly possible for her to have slept, eaten, defecated, and urinated, without any one knowing that she did so.

The conclusions arrived at by M. Warlomont were, that the

stigmatisations and ecstasies of Louise Lateau were real and to be explained upon well-known physiological and pathological principles, that she "worked, and dispensed heat, that she lost every Friday a certain quantity of blood by the stigmata, that the air she expired contained the vapor of water and carbonic acid, that her weight had not materially altered since she had come under observation. She consumes carbon and it is not from her own body that she gets it. Where does she get it from? Physiology answers, 'She eats.'"

Relative to the assumed abstinence in the cases of Palma d'Oria, Louise Lateau and other subjects of ecstasy and stigmata, it is not necessary, in view of the remarks already made on this subject in a previous chapter, to devote further consideration to it here. The conclusion arrived at by M. Warlomont is the only one which science can tolerate. Should Louise Lateau or Palma d'Oria ever be subjected to as close watching as was the poor little Welsh Fasting Girl, Sarah Jacob, it will certainly terminate as badly for them as for her, unless they yield to the demands of nature and take the food which the organism requires.

But a few words in regard to the scientific aspect of the stigmatization will probably not be considered out of place.

The connection between certain affections of the skin and the nervous system, has only been a subject of particular attention during the past ten or twelve years. Now, dermatologists make one of the most important classes of skin diseases to be the direct result of nervous derangement. A very familiar example is the urticaria or hives, so frequently met with, especially in children, as the effect of emotional disturbance.

In the disease known as purpura, the blood is deficient in red corpuscles, while there is an increase in the white globules, a condition of this fluid which the investigations of M. Warlomont showed to exist in the case of Louise Lateau. The affection is further characterized by a tendency of the blood to transude through the coats of the vessels, and in some cases to the formation of aneurismal dilatations of the capillaries, appearing on the surface as little ulcerations, and the rupture of which allows the blood to escape.

Many cases of hæmidrosis, or bloody sweat are scattered through medical treatises, and several monographs have been devoted to the consideration of the subject.

Thus Boerhaave relates the case of a young girl who was subject to the occurence of ampullæ on various parts of her body, from which blood flowed in abundance, and which then, as did those of Palma d'Oria, disappeared without leaving any trace. These hæmorrhages took place very often, and among other places from the right hand, the front of the neck, the right arm and the right leg. She even wept tears of blood, a circumstance not mentioned of any one of the stigmatized mystics, but one calculated still further to excite the astonishment of those on the look-out for miraculous events.

The fact that such hæmorrhages follow closely on the occurrence of any strong emotion is well established. As the counterpart to the cases of Palma d'Oria, Louise Lateau, and other so-called miraculous instances of stigmata, I adduce the following instance from Dr. Magnus Huss of Stockholm, as cited by M. Bourneville.*

* Louise Lateau, ou la Stigmatisée Belge. Paris, 1875, p. 32.

Maria K., a servant girl aged 23, was born in the country, of poor parents. Her father and mother had always been in good health, never having shown any disposition either to hæmorrhages or to affections of the nervous system. The same may be said of the other ancestors of Maria, and of her brothers and sisters.

Maria is of medium height, of lymphatic constitution and presents the appearance of good health. Her skin is delicate, her complexion high colored, her hair brown, almost black, her eyes a grayish blue, her figure full. At fifteen years of age her menstruation began with regularity, and has continued so without any interruption. This fact is to be noted, for M. Lefebvre cites a like circumstance in Louise Lateau as one of the proofs that her case is not to be classed with those of mundane etiology.

In her infancy, Maria suffered from attacks of convulsions, but latterly she has not been ill. Accidental wounds of the skin do not give place to hæmorrhages, and her flesh heals as well as that of other people. At nineteen she went out to service. She asserts that the family with whom she lived treated her badly.

On the 4th of August, 1850, Maria was severely beaten, and was struck with a hard body on the head. These blows, with the anger and fear they provoked, caused convulsions, and she was for half an hour unconscious. When she came to herself she observed that a severe hæmorrhage had occurred from the hairy part of the scalp, and from a place where there had been no wound. During the two following weeks the hæmorrhage from the head continued. Besides, she bled from the eyes, or from the face around the eyes, from the left ear, and finally she vomited blood.

For fifteen days she was better, and then another hæmorrhage from the scalp and stomach took place during her sleep. The hæmorrhage continued for eight days, then it stopped spontaneously, and Maria was in a good state of health for two months. At the end of that period, and following immediately on a strong emotion, she bled from the head, from the borders of the eyelids, and from the left ear. Since then the hæmorrhages were produced regularly at intervals of from eight to fifteen days, and lasted for one or two days. In the intervals, Maria was in good health, although physically weaker than before the beginning of this disease. She had a good appetite, and her bowels were regular. Her menstruation was not only not suspended, but it occurred with perfect regularity, even during the periods of the hæmorrhagic attacks, not being changed either as regarded quantity or duration.

In February and July, 1851, the hæmorrhages appeared at irregular intervals, and were more or less abundant. About the middle of July she was admitted into the Seraphim Hospital in Stockholm, where she was examined successively by Profs. Santessen, Malmessen and Magnus Huss. Aside from the existence of a chloro-anæmic condition, all the organs were in good health, and all the functions regular.

The hæmorrhages often supervened upon emotional disturbance, and at irregular periods. They were in general preceded by an *ensemble* of symptoms which recalled to mind those observed with Louise Lateau—a sensation of pressure or weight on the top of the head, a feeling of vertigo, and of general fatigue, noises in the ears, and frequent pulse. When the exuding surface was examined with a lens no trace of excoriation of the skin was discovered. And even when the hæmorrhage had lasted five or six days, the most careful inspection failed to show any sign of a cicatrix. During the hæmorrhages the region affected was painful to the touch, and the temperature was elevated.

A certain number of attacks (convulsions and hæmorrhages) were complicated with vomiting of blood, with ecchymosis, and apparent bruises on the left half of the body. They were never observed on the right side. The limbs on the left side were always, at the time of the hæmorrhages, semi-paralysed. and the paralysis remained for periods ranging from six days to two or three weeks. Consciousness always returned to her suddenly, as if she had wakened from a long sleep.

"One circumstance," writes Dr. Huss, "nearly twenty years before Louise Lateau had begun to exhibit the stigmata, deserves to be reported in view of its psychological importance. She was not slow to notice that she was the object of particular attention, and that her disease was studied with great curiosity. As among those visiting the hospital, some saw her while the hæmorrhages were present, and others hearing them spoken of, made her presents, often of considerable value, she began, as was very evident, to cause at will the phenomena to take place. And this she did by seeking a quarrel with some other patient, and the excitement into which she was thereby thrown produced the hæmorrhage she desired. It seemed also that she could, without such cause, by the mere effort of her will, throw herself into such a mental condition that the hæmorrhage resulted."

In his very valuable memoir, M. Parrot* distinctly affirms the fact of hæmorrhages of the kind in question. In the case of Louise Lateau the hæmorrhages occurred on Fridays, sometimes, however, missing. The mental excitement produced in her by the devotional contemplation of the events which the Church associates with this day, as well as the exercise of her own will in the matter, are sufficient causes of the periodicity observed in her case. Besides, when the habit had become well established, no other exciting cause would be required than the force resulting from the constant repetition of an act by the organism at some particular time. No one competent to form an opinion after a scientific study of the subject, and not bound in the trammels of a most abject superstition, can fail to see the absolute identity in all essential respects of the cases of Maria K. and Louise Lateau. And this is only one case. Many others are mentioned by M. Parrot, M. Chauffard, Wilson, Mason Good, and dermatologists generally.

One further point only in regard to Louise Lateau. The report of M. Warlomont was made to the Royal Academy of Medicine of Belgium. In the debate which ensued upon the presentation of the report, views were advanced in favor of, and against the miraculous interposition of Providence to produce the stigmata, according to the predilections of the speakers. M. Lefebvre held to his view of miracle in the case, and M. Crocq declared that it did not pass beyond the category of pathological occurrences. And then, after several forms of expression had been proposed, the Academy decided to have

* Etude sur la sueur de sang et les hæmorrhages néuropathiques. Paris, 1859.

nothing further to do with the subject, either in its theological or pathological aspects beyond printing the memoir of M. Charbonnier, who was the first to call attention to the scientific points of the case, and passing a vote of thanks to him for his contribution to its archives.

In the mean time Louise Lateau continues her ecstasies and stigmatizations, and many will continue to regard them as miraculous, no matter how thoroughly her pretensions are exposed; and while she can gain notoriety by acting the crucifixion every Friday, it is very certain, unless she wearies of the monotony, that she will keep up the habit she has established.

CHAPTER XVII.

CONCLUSION.

And this concludes what I have to say now, relative to the important subjects which have been under consideration. It would be very easy to extend the inquiry much further, and in other directions, and at some future time I may be tempted to do so. My main object has been to show that so far as the matters which have engaged our attention are concerned, there are no phenomena connected with them which are not readily explainable by well-known physiological, pathological, or physical laws, and that many assertions made in reference to them are fraudulent and false.

We see, too, that at all times during the historic period two classes of individuals have been concerned in the propagation of false ideas relative to certain phenomena which have been regarded as supernatural. These are the deceivers and the deceived. Whether as priests, witches, magicians, mesmerizers, somnambulists, ecstatics, hysterical persons, or mediums—the first are deceivers, some of them honest, but by far the greater number guilty of intentional fraud. Whether subject to illusions, hallucinations, or delusions; whether weak-minded, superstitious, or ignorant—the second are deceived.

In the foregoing pages I have attempted among other things to give an outline view of some of the causes which produce many so-called supernatural manifestations, and which lead to their acceptance by certain classes of individuals. To describe, in detail, all the vagaries of spiritualism would be a fruitless undertaking. I have witnessed many spiritualistic performances, and have never seen a single one which could not be accounted for by the operation of some one or more of the causes specified. No medium has ever yet been lifted into the air by spirits no one has ever read unknown writing through a closed envelope, no one has ever lifted tables or chairs but by material agencies, no one has ever been tied or untied by spirits, no one has ever heard the knock of a spirit, and no one has ever spoken through the power of a spirit other than his own.

Even if bodies had been raised in the air by agencies unexplainable, even if some one had read writing through several thicknesses of paper, even if others had been bound and unbound in a way unknown to us, even if knocks had been heard whose sources could not be ascertained, even if the causes of all the phenomena of spiritualism were entirely beyond our present knowledge, there would be no proof that spirits had any thing to do with them. On the contrary, the hypothesis of spirits is altogether the least plausible which could be suggested. The phenomena and the explanation have nothing in common.

Spiritualism is a religion. As such it is held tenaciously and honestly by many well-meaning people. To reason with these would be a waste of words, just as much as would be the attempt to persuade a madman out of his delusion. Emotion or interest or accident might change them, but facts never. But there are some who halt between belief and unbelief, for the reason mainly that they have no clear conception of what knowledge is, and of how things are to be proved. For these there can be no more striking truths than the following account of Algazzali's description of his search for actual knowledge:

"The true source of casual beliefs is the authority of parents and preceptors. Now, there are many methods of comprehending the differences which exist between things received on the faith of such authority and the principles of the things themselves. There exist likewise many means of distinguishing the true from the false. For this reason I said to myself in the very beginning of my inquiry, 'My object is simply to know the truth of things, consequently it is indispensable to seek for that which constitutes knowledge.' Now, it is evident to me that certain knowledge ought to be that which explains the object to be known, so that there can be no doubt, and that all error and all conjecture would be henceforth impossible. And not only then the understanding would not need to make efforts to arrive at certainty, but the security against error ought to be in so intimate a connection with the thing known for certain, that even when an apparent proof of its falsity is produced—as, for example, if a man should transform a stone into gold or a stick into a serpent—no error should be caused, or even the suspicion of error rendered possible. If, when I have satisfied myself that ten is more than three, some one should say to me, 'Not so, on the contrary three is more than ten, and to prove to you the truth of my assertion I will transform this rod into a snake;' if then he should so transform it to my entire convic tion, the certainty I should have of his error would not be shaken. His performance would produce in me only an admiration for his skill, but I should not doubt the truth I had acquired.

"Then I was convinced that all knowledge which I did not possess in this manner, and of which I had not this kind of certitude, could inspire me with neither confidence nor assurance, and that all knowledge without assurance is not a sure knowledge."*

How little the phenomena of spiritualism are reconcilable with the tests laid down by Algazzali, every candid, intelligent, and educated inquirer knows.

* Essai sur les Ecoles philosophiques chez les Arabes et notamment sur la Doctrine d'Algazzali. Par Auguste Schmölders, Docteur en Philosophie Paris, 1842.

Made in the USA
Monee, IL
04 November 2026

67391585R00213